FITNESS OVER 50

Complete Step-by-Step Guide to Become Lean, Muscular and In the Best Shape Ever With an Exact Weekly Workout Plan

Stanford Dyson

Copyright ©, Stanford Dyson

TABLE OF CONTENTS

INTRODUCTION

How to be in the Best Shape Ever – After the Age of 50

Congratulations on purchasing *Fitness Over 50,* and thank you for doing so.

The following chapters will discuss how you can be in the best shape ever – after the age of 50.   Failing to stay in shape as you age can predispose you to obesity, increasing your risk factors for heart disease and diabetes. These increase your chance of loss of memory and other cognition skills that are the real fear factors of aging.

You *can* age gracefully. You can maintain a youthful façade – both physically and mentally. How? Exercise is the key. A healthy diet is its helpmate.

Think of this book as the master lock and key to your continuing youthfulness. It will give you the guidance you need to be in the best shape possible, whether you've neglected your body for years or you're trying to maintain what you've always considered your sacred temple.

In these pages, you'll find the three most important exercises to a quick, full-body workout. You'll learn how and when to increase weight or distance. You'll understand how to prevent injury. And how to recover if the unfortunate should occur.

You'll learn how to eat your way to health to maintain a youthful physique. You'll also learn that a guide like this can be your best friend. You may even want to share it – but only with a best friend you trust won't steal your woman 'cause these tips will make any man an animal even after he's passed the big 5-O.

There are plenty of books on this subject on the market. This is the one you're going to keep. Thanks again for choosing this one! Every effort was made to ensure it is full of as much useful information as possible. Please enjoy!

CHAPTER 1: FITNESS FOR EVERYONE

Why Exercise Is Essential to Good Health

Hopefully, you've stayed fit, and this will be addressing the changes your body has made now that you're over 50. Maybe you've neglected yourself, and you need to *re-start* a fitness routine – 'cause now you've hit the big 5-0! Maybe you've never had to exercise before, but now that you've hit that number that you can't deny is on the downhill slide, you know you can't avoid it anymore. It's time to EXERCISE!

Don't Worry: It's not as bad as you think. Fitness doesn't have to be a chore – no matter how old you are or your current physical state. You're going to find tips and techniques here that will help working out feel like fun.

Exercise is essential to your good health. After 50, it becomes harder to rein in your physical fitness, if you've neglected it. Not impossible, just harder. The benefits become more and more crucial.

After 50, weight gain becomes more prevalent. We tend to gain weight at a rate of about 1 to 2 pounds per year every year past the age of 30. That's as much as 40 pounds by the time we're 50. And we're going to keep packing them on.

What contributes to that weight gain? After age 30 (again), muscle starts to turn to fat if you don't work it. That accelerates at age 60, so you really want to combat that in these last years before you meet that age marker. Fat requires less energy for the body to operate than muscle. If you don't take in fewer calories to compensate for the lower energy requirements, you gain weight.

Fat *turnover* (how quickly fat is removed from your body) also slows with age. But exercise – particularly strength training or resistance exercises – helps to stimulate your muscles. To maintain muscle, you need to eat a higher protein diet as well.

Another contributor to weight increase with age is that testosterone that regulates muscle mass and fat distribution begins to drop at around 40 years of age.

What else increases weight with age? Lower muscle mass often contributes to a more sedentary lifestyle with aging. Stress increases cortisol that increases body fat. Metabolism slows and becomes less efficient. Again, strength training can help compensate for all three of these.

Another important reason to exercise is that it boosts your mood. No matter what your situation in life, being in a better mood is a benefit. Exercise helps with that.

Whether you're currently practicing good health and fitness, or you need to start from a sedentary lifestyle, it's time to assess your current fitness level.

How to Assess Your Current Fitness Level

Getting a Physical

- It's time to see your doctor for a physical. If you are already in a physical fitness program, it's a good time to assess your fitness level. If you are not, it's time to see what your limitations are.
- Are you at a healthy weight? Should you gain/lose weight?
- How's your blood pressure?

Normal blood pressure is 120 or less over 80 or less. If your blood pressure is 130 over 80 or higher, you have hypertension. Discuss this condition with your doctor and decided whether it is safe for you to proceed with an exercise program or not. And what, if any, precautions you should take.

- Your heart rate should be between 50 and 100, though many healthy people have slower heart rates.
- Respiration rate is considered normal with breaths that are 12 to 16 per minute. Twenty breaths per minute might mean a heart or lung problem that your doctor will discuss with you. Be sure to ask whether or not it is safe for you to proceed with an exercise program and how you should modify it, if necessary.
- Your doctor will listen to your heart for an irregular beat, a murmur, or any other signs of heart disease. These may also be indicated by blood testing.
- Your lungs, too, will be listened to for crackles, wheezes, or other indications of lung disease.
- A routine head and neck exam will be performed to view your eyes, ears, nose, throat, sinuses, lymph nodes, thyroid, and carotid arteries.
- The abdominal exam will help detect your liver size, presence of abdominal fluid, or tenderness, and a stethoscope will help listen for bowel sounds.
- Your doctor will also test your reflexes, balance, mental state, nerves, and muscle strength ("squeeze my finger as tight as you can").
- A skin exam should be included in your physical, and this includes an examination of your nails.

- Your joints and extremities will be examined for good pulsation and any possible abnormalities. Arthritis may be setting in by this age.
- During your testicular exam, your doctor can check for lumps, tenderness, or changes in size. Most men notice a cancerous growth before seeing their doctor.
- A hernia exam is when your doctor will say, 'turn your head and cough" while checking for abdominal wall weakness between the intestines and the scrotum.
- A penis exam can reveal warts or ulcers or other evidence of sexually transmitted infection.
- By inserting a finger in the rectum, your doctor can examine your prostate for the correct size and shape.
- In addition to the physical examination, lab tests may be ordered to include complete blood count, chemistry panel, and urinalysis.
- If you haven't had one in a while (recommendation is every 4 – 6 years), a lipid panel may be ordered to check cholesterol levels for an increased chance of stroke or heart attack.
- Blood sugar is more likely to be checked if you are overweight or have diabetes risk factors, though the American Diabetes Association recommends all adults over age 45 – regardless of weight –have it checked.
- Once you turn 50, you should begin having regular colorectal cancer screenings. If you have immediate family members who had it or you have other risk factors, that screening should be started sooner.
- If you smoke, drink heavily, or have any other chronic health issues, be certain you have discussed these and your intention to exercise with your doctor before you leave his office.

How to Begin a Fitness Program

The hardest part of beginning a fitness program is taking the first step. It will continue to be difficult until you've made it a routine. By visiting your doctor and assessing your 'fitness,' you've taken the first step. Beginning to move is your hardest *second* step.

A healthy fitness program needs to include the following elements:

- Healthy diet
- Cardio/Aerobics
- Strength training

When all of these are included and performed correctly, injuries will be prevented.

Aerobics refers to oxygen intake. Cardio refers to the heart. When you're doing aerobics, you will be getting cardio.

Aerobics is an easy place to begin because it does not have to be as strenuous as it sounds. You remember aerobics as being Jane Fonda shaking her beauteous booty in leotards that left nothing to the imagination. You remember it as the beginning of the jogging fad – which became a phenomenon that proved to be anything but a fad. You remember it as Richard Simmons 'Sweating to the Oldies'.

That was then: this is now. What we've learned is that aerobics doesn't have to be as strenuous as all that. The requirement necessary for an activity to be cardio is that it elevates your heartbeat. Therefore, gardening qualifies as cardio/aerobic activity. That is unless all you're doing is deadheading flowers. Sorry, folks, that's not aerobic.

But if you're bending down, picking several handfuls of weeds, turning around and placing them a couple of steps away in a wheelbarrow, and doing this fast enough to up your breathing rate, you're working aerobically.

Take a brisk walk – at about 2.5 miles per hour. You're working aerobically. You're getting a cardio workout. Generally, you can tell you are working aerobically because you can just barely carry on a conversation. You will have to pause your speaking more often than normal to suck in a breath.

The American Heart Association workout guidelines recommend 150 minutes per week of moderate-intensity or 75 minutes per week of vigorous-intensity aerobic activity per week or a combination of both plus moderate- to high-intensity strength training at least two times per week. These minutes should be spread out over the entire week. It's important to note that strength training is recommended *at least* two times per week. Since you are now over 50 and losing muscle to age, you can easily increase that to 3 times per week.

Moderate-intensity aerobics include:

- Brisk walking or hiking
- Water aerobics or slow swimming
- Dancing
- Doubles Tennis
- Biking slower than 10 miles/hour
- Gardening

Vigorous aerobics include:

- Jogging or running
- Swimming laps
- Aerobic dance
- Hiking up a hill or with a heavy backpack
- Cycling faster than 10 miles per hour

- Jumping Rope
- Heavy Yard Work (Digging or hoeing)

Use your target heart rate as a guide. You got this at the doctor during your physical, remember? 50-100 beats per minute (bpm) is normal. If you're an athlete or more active, it will be lower. Stress, anxiety, medications, and hormones can increase it.

Your *maximum* heart rate is 220 minus your age. So if you just turned 50, your maximum heart rate is 170. Your *target* heart rate – the rate you want to hit during moderate activity – is 50-70% of that rate and 70-85% of that rate during intense physical activity.

Here's a chart to show you your target heart rate zone and your maximum heart rate:

AGE	Target HR Zone 50-85%	Average Maximum HR 100%
50 years	85-145 bpm	170 bpm
55 years	83-140 bpm	165 bpm
60 years	80-136 bpm	160 bpm
65 years	78-132 bpm	155 bpm
70 years	75-128 bpm	150 bpm

Try to hit the target zone while you're doing your aerobic activity without hitting the maximum. When you hit the maximum, that's your signal that you *need to slow down*. That's why it's called the maximum. Consider it as the yellow light right before a heart attack.

See Chapter 2: Cardio/Aerobics for workout suggestions.

How to Make Your Fitness Program a Routine

It is essential that your fitness program become a routine. You need to work out six days a week, allowing yourself one day a week of rest. You need to vary your workout program to avoid boredom. Part of the way you will do that is by including 2 – 3 days of strength training per week. Here are some ideas to make your fitness program a routine.

- **Same time every day** – If you work out at the same time every day, it is more likely to become a routine – like brushing your teeth or eating breakfast or getting up. You know how you set your alarm for 8 am every day, but after a while, you start to wake up a few minutes *before* the alarm goes off? That's what it will become like with your workout routine. Your body will start to anticipate the exercise if you do it at the same time every day.
- **Workout reminder** – Set your phone alarm to go off at the same time every day to remind you to go work out. Maybe you need two alarms: one that tells you it's time to get ready and one that tells you 'start working out.'
- **Message on lock screen** - Set up a message on your lock screen that says, "Work Out Today." This is especially helpful if you have an inconsistent schedule that prevents you from working out at the same time every day, but you can fit it in when time allows. Remember that the American Heart Association workout guidelines recommend 150 minutes per week of moderate-intensity or 75 minutes per week of vigorous-intensity aerobic activity per week or a combination of both plus moderate- to high-intensity strength training at least two times per week. These minutes should be spread out over the entire week.
  - o You do not have to have more than 15 or 20 minutes at a time to get in a good workout. The faster you are, the less time you need. In fact, you can combine your strength training with

aerobic activity. The full-body workout thruster is a strength training move that, when done quickly, becomes aerobic. There are numerous other aerobic strength training moves listed in Chapter 3: Strength Training>Body Weight Resistance>Cardio/Aerobic Body Weight Resistance Suggested Workouts.

- **Partner Up** – Working with a partner comes with responsibility. Your partner will depend on you to show up for the workout, and if you don't, you are letting them down. Ahhh, the guilt! That just might be the encouragement you need to keep your workout going strong.

- **Build a community** – Get to know someone at the gym. Make it social. When you walk into the gym, and people greet you by name, it often gives the warm, friendly feeling needed to want to get there as often as possible. If socializing is important to you, then this may just the kind of atmosphere you need. If recognition of your effort is important, this is another reason to build a community. Other people at the gym may start to count on seeing you there and say, "Hey, I missed you on Tuesday," when you're not there. That will encourage you not to miss a single workout.

- **Ditch the Win or Lose Attitude** – A little exercise is better than none. So if today isn't a great workout, or – Oops! – you didn't work out at all. That doesn't mean you blew it. You can pick it back up tomorrow, and you are still working out. You don't have to 'go back to the beginning.' It's not Monopoly, 'Go directly to jail. Do not pass. Do not collect $200.' Nope. There's no punishment but your own guilt, and when you workout tomorrow, that will be all gone, and you will have the high that comes with the adrenalin of working out. It's a win-win all over again.

- **Realistic Expectations** – Don't try to run 10 miles your first day out. In fact, for most people, even five miles is too much. Walk at a fast pace (2.5 miles/hour) for two miles if you've been sedentary and haven't had a steady workout routine recently. Guidelines are in Chapter 2: Cardio/Aerobics.

- o Don't expect to lift unrealistic weights. You will make yourself sore, and then you won't be able to work out the next day. Your goal is to be able to continue a consistent, regular exercise program. Overdoing your workout sessions will only discourage you and prevent you from further exercise. You want your workout routine to become just that – routine. So making it realistic is essential.

- o Apply this to your weight goals as well. Don't expect to gain or lose your weight goals in a week. Don't expect to change the shape of your body in a week. Allow at least four weeks of consistency to begin to *see* your results. Once the visual encouragement begins, continuing your routine becomes easier. By then, your workouts have pretty much become a routine already.

- **Variety** – Mix it up, be creative, use variety. Doing the same workout day after day will become dull. It is the number one reason for gym dropout. Change up your routine. If you regularly jog, try hiking up the hill. If you regularly swim, try something you've never done before, say, climbing or mountain biking or spinning class.

  - o If you regularly use free weights, try a whole strength training session of bodyweight resistance only. There is an endless variety of strength training exercises. Boredom is never an excuse here.

- **Keep a Journal** – Keeping a journal helps you keep track of exactly how long your workout was last week, how much you were lifting, how far you walked or ran, how many laps you swam. You can also use it to keep track of your diet.

  - o Note any changes. Note your goals. Highlight your accomplishments. That way, you have a visual incentive at a glance. If you have a bad workout, note it too. There may be a pattern. Perhaps Saturday morning after Friday night's drinking is not a good day for a run, for example. Your workout journal can help you spot these trends.

- **Listen to music** – There's nothing like a great tune to keep you motivated to move during your workout. Music can change your whole attitude. If you didn't feel like working out while you were putting on your workout clothes, once you start hearing the music, you will suddenly feel yourself wanting to move, wanting to stretch your muscles, wanting to just *groove*. I know you know what I mean!

To find some great workout grooves, just search one of the following:

- Warm-up playlist
- Pump up songs
- Slow workout playlist
- Walking music playlist
- Workout playlist
- Treadmill Songs
- Motivational Running Songs
- High-Energy Cardio Mix
- Aerobic Cardio Dance Workout
- Jogging & Running Music
- Clean Workout Music
- Pissed off Workout playlist
- 180 BMP Running Workout Mix
- After Workout Music
- Cool Down Music
- Chillhop Radio
- Slow Music – For example, prepare some slow music for your Cool Down After Working Out
- Amazing Music for Stretching

- Stretching Music Set
- Music for Stretching
- Workout Cool down Playlist
- Fitness Calming Down Stretching Music Mix

CHAPTER 2: CARDIO/AEROBICS

Don't You Dare Skip This Chapter!

It's tempting to skip right past this chapter because you think this is going to be tough. But if you thoroughly read the last chapter, then you know that cardio/aerobics does not have to be strenuous to start. Below are the outlines for a beginner or introductory cardio/aerobic workout as well as how to move into the more advanced workout and how to work at an athletic level cardio/aerobic capacity.

If you are already in a workout program, skip right to your current level.

What Is Cardio/Aerobics?

Cardio means the heart, and aerobics means oxygen uptake. Getting your heart beating with cardio puts you into an aerobic state of pumping oxygen.

Warm-Up

Before any workout, do a warm-up. Your warm-up starts the blood flowing to your muscles to increase your range of motion and decrease muscle tension and pain. This is the beginning of your injury prevention routine.

Since you are no longer a spring chicken, your joints need to be part of your warm-up routine. This can be done on your way to wherever you are going to work out. All you need to do is get the synovial fluid moving through your joints by manipulating them. Synovial fluid is what lubricates your joints into moving smoothly. Think of this as working arthritis out of your joints.

You're going to move every joint in your body from your neck down to your toes. Perform about ten movements in each direction on every joint. These can be done while you're walking or driving.

Joint Warm-Up

> **Neck**: Drop your head forward. Rotate to the right. Drop forward. Rotate to the left. Now, do it again but in change direction.
>
> Gently drop your head back. Rotate towards your right shoulder. Return to center. Rotate towards your left shoulder. Switch your direction.
>
> Full neck rotation: Start at your right shoulder and rotate all the way to the left, drop your head to the back and rotate all the way to your right shoulder. Perform about three rotations. Change the direction.
>
> **Shoulders**: Roll your shoulders backward, isolating them. Nothing else needs to move but your shoulders. Do both at once. Switch your direction. You want to perform about ten circles in each direction.
>
> **Elbows**: Hold your arms out to the sides and allow your arms to hang down like a puppet. Rotate them both towards your body. After ten rotations, turn them away from your body. Your upper arms should remain still.
>
> **Wrists**: Rotate your wrists – this is easiest if you form your hands into fists. If you're driving, please do one hand at a time. Otherwise, do both at once, rotating hands towards each other for ten turns and then away for the same number of turns.

Fingers: Wiggle all your fingers at once as though they were spiders going crazy. Keep this up for at least 30 seconds.

Trunk Rotations: Stand with feet hip-width apart. Bend forward from the waist – this will not be a deep bend but a slightly leaning forward. You are only warming up, not stretching, simply moving synovial fluid through your spine. Lean a little to the left, to the back, to the right. Return to the front and begin another rotation.

Hip Rotations: This one's easy and feels pretty good. Simply thrust your hips forward and rotate around – left, back, right. Then reverse direction. Be sure you do at least ten in each direction.

Knee Rotation: Be gentle here. Lift your knee and allow your calf to hang loosely down. Gently swivel your calf in circles till you've completed ten rotations. You may have to pause after five, switch legs, then return to the original leg for the last five. Go to the opposite leg to perform reverse rotations and continue switching legs until you've performed ten rotations in each direction.

Ankle Rotations: This is easy, folks. Just stick your ankle out and rotate. Do at least ten in each direction. This is going to get all that synovial fluid flowing into the joint in your ankle and prepare you for a nice workout.

Toes: You can't exactly rotate your toes. Instead, just scrunch and stretch until you've done ten for each foot.

Dynamic Warm-Up: Now is the time to warm-up your muscles for the workout ahead. Dynamic warm-ups are directly related to the intended exercise. If your workout is a jog, a good dynamic workout is a slow and easy jog for about five minutes until your muscles begin to feel warm and move easily. Then move into your full running workout.

If you're doing a bike ride, you might want to start with leg lifts or high knee lift marching in the same place without moving. Again, for about five minutes until the blood really begins to flow to those large muscles before jumping on your bike.

All warmed up? Let's move to the workouts.

Be sure to drink plenty of water while you are working out, and to try to reach, but not exceed, your target heart rate. Check it frequently as you exercise.

Beginning Cardio/Aerobics Workout

Less strenuous than you think and still benefits the heart. Be sure you've done your joint rotations so that synovial fluid is flowing in all of your joints. Do a dynamic warm-up that is appropriate for the cardio/aerobic workout of your choice. Then you're ready to start in on your first workout.

As a beginner, you will be taking it slow. There's no need to strain. Your goal is 150 minutes of moderate aerobic activity for the week. We're going to break that down to 4 -37 ½ minute workouts per week. You're going to use two days a week for strength training and take one day a week off.

Don't worry if you don't have 37 ½ minutes all at once. You can break that down to 18 ¾ minutes twice a day. That's about how long it takes to walk your dog. And he does need to go out at least twice a day. Walking the dog, by the way, is an excellent time to do body-resistance exercises as covered in Chapter 3: Strength Training. If you spread your body resistance exercises over the whole week, that gives you two extra days to do your cardio/aerobics. That means you only need to do 25 minutes per day or 12 ½ minutes twice a day. Even a really busy schedule can fit in 12 ½ minutes twice a day.

Remember your target heart rate and try to reach but not exceed it.

Some of your beginner options for working out include:

- Try brisk walking, where you're walking at a brisk pace (2.5 miles per hour). You should be aiming to be able to talk but not sing. A good dynamic warm-up (after your joint warm-ups) would be slow marching in the same place without moving, with high knee lifts for about five minutes just until your blood is flowing warmly through your body and your beginning to feel increased breathing. Be sure to keep your march slow so that you don't elevate your heart rate too high. This is only a warm-up.
- Hiking. The terrain should no longer be flat but not uphill as you are only a beginner, and we do not want this to be such a strenuous exercise session that you either become sore for days or become so winded that you exceed your target heart rate.
  - A good dynamic hiking warm-up (after your joint warm-ups) is to quickly perform side lunges switching side to side about ten times, front lunges switching legs fairly rapidly about ten times, and about ten bodyweight squats. These will bring your body temperature up and start increasing your breathing, preparing you for your cardio/aerobic hike.
- Dance. Because you are in the beginning stages of your health and fitness, you should choose something with a moderate – not fast – tempo. "Crazy for You" by Madonna comes to mind. Use a swaying motion keeping your arms down and your feet mostly on the floor. If you are not reaching your target heart rate, you may lift your legs a bit higher or begin to lift your arms. Stay aware of your breathing. You are aiming to be able to talk but not sing.

Singers who dance while they are singing are in *excellent* physical condition. You are not in that cardio/aerobic condition – yet!

- o Just dancing itself is a good dynamic warm-up (after joint warm-ups). Begin slowly with moderate side to side steps, building pace and endurance. For quick warming of muscles, try marching in the same place without moving, with high slow leg raises for about five minutes before you start to dance at your target heart rate.

- Calisthenics. If you choose this one, move slowly. You are a beginner. These are body resistance exercises that will strengthen your muscles while giving you a cardio/aerobic workout. You will pause and walk when you feel winded or pass your target heart rate. See Chapter 3: Strength Training>Body Weight Resistance for specific suggestions.

- o A good dynamic warm-up (after your joint warm-ups) is to quickly perform side lunges switching side to side about ten times, front lunges switching legs fairly rapidly about ten times, and about ten bodyweight squats. These will bring your body temperature up and start increasing your breathing, preparing you for your cardio/aerobic calisthenics.

- Treadmill. 2.5 miles per hour with no incline for your full workout period.

- o Most treadmills have a programable warm-up. Perform a joint warm-up before beginning the treadmill cycle, then use the treadmill's warm-up and workout cycles. Be sure to use a workout that fits into the parameters of your fitness level and stay within your target heart rate zone.

- Slow swimming. Be sure you monitor your breathing. You should be able to speak but not sing. Swim either with your head above water or keep your head up long enough at the end of each lap to check your breathing or target heart rate to make sure you are on track and not exceeding your maximum. Remember also not to push too hard. This one is easy to overdo, and you do not want to be sore for days afterward as that will simply cause discouragement.

- o Be certain you have performed joint warm-ups before you begin your workout. As a dynamic warm-up, consider jogging in the same place without moving while you are in the pool. This will be slow going as the water resists your movement but your muscles will start to warm-up, and your breathing will become elevated. Be sure you remain within your target heart rate zone during your entire workout, including the warm-up.
- Slow bike ride. Riding a bike uses your biggest muscles – your thighs. Therefore, it quickly puts you in a cardio/aerobic state. Be certain you monitor your breathing (you should be able to speak but not sing) and target heart rate. Do not exceed these limits. You want to be safe and avoid injury. Keep it slow and steady.
  - o After your joint warm-up, do a dynamic warm-up for your bike ride of a slow marching in the same place without moving, with high knee lifts. This uses the same large thigh, hamstring, and glute muscles you will use for riding your bike and allows the blood to start flowing into these muscles while elevating your breathing.
- These are not the only activities you can do for your beginner workout. But they are a good foundation. Be sure to change up your activity for variety so that you remain interested in working out. You do not have to do a new activity every day, only often enough to alleviate your boredom.

Building Your Heart Muscle for Longevity – When to Increase Capacity

Your body will quickly adapt to your workout. It will become easier and easier. Yet, you will have a psychological barrier. Somedays, working out will feel like *such* a chore. But your body will find it easier and easier to pump the blood through your heart and muscles and process the oxygen through your lungs. Just keep your mind strong. You'll adapt. Read the tips and tricks in the next section for ways to keep yourself moving forward.

When it's no longer difficult for you to talk at your current level of exercise, and when you are at the bottom of or under your target heart rate, it's time to increase your cardio/aerobic level. You are ready for a new challenge. Move up to the next level.

Advanced Cardio/Aerobics Workout

Here are a few ways to get yourself into the zone for your new – harder – workout:

- **Be Silly** – Whether in public or in private, try something silly, like a quick maniac dance that energizes your body and soul and prepares you to kick ass!
- **Pay Attention to Your Diet** – Most athletes prefer to perform on an empty stomach but in the days leading up to your increased capacity, pay special attention to your diet, and increase your Omega-3s. These can have the effect of easing your tension and relaxing muscles. This way, they are less likely to be inflamed.
- **Re-read Your Journal** – Remind yourself how very far you've come. See that this is simply the next step in what you've already done. This is progress. This is where you are supposed to go. You've been taking baby steps, and this is just another baby step along the path.
- **Visualization** – Following right along on that thought, visualize yourself taking that step. Visualize yourself succeeding. See yourself starting this run (or swim, or uphill climb, or bike ride, etc.), see yourself taking the journey in stride as though you've done it many times fully conditioned. See yourself completing it successfully with comfortable breath and a good target heart rate.

- Visualize your successful workout the night before just as you are about to go to sleep.
- This visualization combines with the Mantra Chant below: Visualize yourself as a machine. You no longer have fragile human parts. You are made of unbreakable titanium. You have no feelings. You are a machine. You have hydraulic pumps for legs and joints. Repeat it. "I am a machine." You feel nothing. Say it. "I feel nothing. I am a machine." Visualize it. You are an unbreakable machine. Your hydraulics pump harder and faster. Repeat it. "I am a machine. I feel nothing. I am unbreakable." Mean it. Say it. Repeat it. Mean it.

- **Chant Positive Mantras** – With each step (pedal, stroke, whatever comes with your exercise), chant a positive mantra like "I got this." Here are a few examples you might repeat:
    - I am strong
    - One more step
    - Keep moving
    - I am a machine.
    - I am unbreakable.
    - I am invincible
    - I can do this.
    - Live like you were dying. (Yes, I'm listening to Tim McGraw as I write this.)
- **Reward Yourself** – Consider laying out a reward for yourself to accept at the end of your workout. A new workout outfit. Dark chocolate. The scenic ride home. A long drink of your favorite wine (which is good for you, by the way. See Chapter 6: Diet.)
- **Find a Motivator** – Check out YouTube for short clips of inspiring athletes like David Goggins (such a badass!) and his 'poopy pants mentality' or Ronnie Coleman, 'lightweight, baby,' one of the greatest bodybuilders of all time. Watch him do a few curls, and you'll know what lifting is all about. These people

overcame obstacles. They didn't start out as super athletes. They started as regular people and worked their way up.

David Goggins went from a broke, overweight exterminator to world-class, Guinness World Record-setting Navy SEAL while fighting past one obstacle after another. You just have to read his story. It's inspiring. Find it at https://www.blogs.va.gov/VAntage/77222/david-goggins-seal-endurance-athlete/ or listen to it on YouTube. His successes came once he endured numerous hardships. Let him teach you not to let your hardships set you back.

Maybe you need motivation from someone a little closer to your age. I get that. So here are a few memorable athletes (since we're talking health and fitness here) over 50:

- Herschel Walker is 51. He was an NFL running back. Now he's an MMA fighter. Can you believe that? If he can step into the ring, you can jog for 20 minutes, then pump some iron.
- In 2008, Ken Mink was the oldest person ever to score in a college Basketball game (Roane State Community College versus King College). At 78, he still plays basketball – against kids in their 20s!
- Morgan Shepherd became the second-oldest NASCAR race *winner* (after Harry Grant) in 1993 at the age of 51 years, four months, and 27 days and he holds the record for the oldest driver to start a race (2014 Spring Cup).
- 1983 Bears draft pick Willie Gault, turned to 100 and 200-meter dashes in his 50s. He set the world record for the 100 meters in the 50 and older age group and the 55 and older age group. Wow!

- Fauja Singh took up long-distance running just over a decade ago at the age of 91 and has completed nine marathons since then. How old are you?

At the Advanced level of intensity, the American Heart Association says you only need 75 minutes per week of aerobic activity plus your two days of strength training per week. That's just 18 ¾ minutes for four days. You'll be taking one day of rest per week.

You'll know you're in the vigorous workout zone because you'll get warm and begin to sweat. You won't be able to talk much without getting out of breath.

As with the Beginning Cardio/Aerobics Workout, the Advanced Cardio Aerobics Workout will begin with a Warm-Up, including the Joint Warm-Up the same as for the beginner workout and the Dynamic Warm-Up with mostly the same guidelines as for the beginner workout.

Be sure to drink plenty of water while working out and try to reach, but not exceed, your target heart rate.

You have prepared yourself for an increase in cardio/aerobic activity. Now psyche yourself up. This will be more difficult than your last workout. Put on your best workout music. Let's get psyched. Go for it!

Ready? Set. **Workout!**

Some of the workout options for an Advanced Cardio/Aerobics Workout are:

- Hike up a hill or with a heavy backpack. Be sure to hit your target heart rate.
- Go for a run. You should be moving at around six mph (although if your legs are short, this may be slower).

- Swim laps. Don't swim slowly here. Put your face in the water and swim like you're in the Olympics.
- Aerobic dancing.
- Tennis singles.
- Jump rope. Remember that you want to work out for 18 ¾ minutes. Jump rope burns a lot of calories. Ten minutes of jumping rope is equal to 30 minutes of running. You can use a weighted rope to add intensity to your workout for a better all-0ver body workout. You can even download apps to lead you through a workout to help you switch it up and that way, you don't get bored with the standard feet together, both jumping at the same time jump. Here are a couple of other jumps you might want to try:
    - Alternate Foot Step: This is when you jump one foot and then the other – almost like you're walking or running over the rope. This is the step you want to use if you want to go fast.
    - Jump Rope High Knees: This is the Alternate Foot Step with knees lifted high on each step.
    - Jump Rope Mummy Kicks: This is easy – it's another variation on the Alternate Foot Step. Keep your legs straight like a mummy and kick them out alternately as you jump over the rope.
    - Jump Rope Boxer Step Jump: This is an efficient step that lets you go for a long time for cardio conditioning – just like a boxer needs to do. This is an in-place step touch while jumping over the rope.
    - Jump Rope Jacks: Your feet move in and out like in jumping jacks while you jump over the rope between bounces.
    - Jump Rope Criss Cross: This is a basic Jump, but your arms are going to cross in front of you and then back out. You can then change your foot skills with alternate

footsteps, high knees, mummy kicks, boxer step, while still crisscrossing your arms.

- Jump Rope Side Swing: This is less about jumping rope than about looking fancy. Again, this one you can alternate with other jumping rope styles. This will work your upper body more – especially if you're using a weighted rope. You will swirl the rope at your side in a circle, switching sides. You can even crisscross the rope across your body switching hands. You can also put the ends of the rope in each hand and swing hands together as you cross from side to side. You can stand still or jump while you're doing this. This is fun, fun, fun. You are, of course, getting a much better workout when you bounce.
- Backward Jumping: The same jump as the basic jump or Alternate Foot Step, only you will be swinging the rope from the front of your body to the back of your body before jumping over it.
- Try as many styles of jumping as you can. Have at!
- Cycle at ten mph or faster.
- Try your hand at some hard yardwork like digging or hoeing. Mucking horse stalls, hauling hay, or raking hay. Pretty much all barn work will get you into a cardio/aerobic state. Be sure to continually check your target heart rate zone. Many a farmer has collapsed while doing everyday farm work because he went well past the target zone right into – and right past – the maximum heart rate zone. Don't do that.
- Rock climbing. Be sure to use all the right equipment, play safe, and let someone know where you are and what you're doing. Or do it indoors. Take breaks as necessary to stay within your target heart rate zone. Remember that you won't be able to talk much, but you won't be just gasping for air. If you find that you are, slow down.

- Calisthenics - These are body resistance exercises that will strengthen your muscles while giving you a cardio/aerobic workout. See Chapter 3: Strength Training>Body Weight Resistance for specific suggestions. Take breaks as necessary to stay within your target heart rate zone. Remember that you won't be able to talk much, but you won't be just gasping for air. If you find that you are, slow down.

- Treadmill. Include incline and decline to intensify your workout and make it like a hike. Remember, you should be at a pace in which you can't talk much without getting out of breath and that you need to hit and maintain your target heart rate. If you find that you are exceeding it, slow down. Most treadmills have built-in warm-ups and cool-downs. Be sure to do the joint warm-up before you get started on the treadmill, then follow one of the built-in programs so long as you reach your target heart-rate zone. Be sure you do not exceed your maximum heart rate zone.

- Play basketball or soccer, handball, racquetball, or squash. Take breaks as necessary to stay within your target heart rate zone. Remember that you won't be able to talk much, but you won't be just gasping for air. If you find that you are, slow down. Use proper safety equipment, and be sure that you actively play for at least 18 ¾ consecutive minutes to count it as your cardio/aerobic workout. Otherwise, you will need to incorporate another activity. Remember to do your joint warm-up and a dynamic warm-up before beginning the sport. Calisthenics is a good choice before most competitive sports.

- Parkour – This is the act of moving through your environment in as straight a line as possible by going over and through your environment by using the obstacles in your path to jump, swing, and vault your way across the landscape. Take breaks as necessary to stay within your target heart rate zone. Remember that you won't be able to talk much, but you won't be just gasping for air. If you find that you are, slow down. As with all cardio/aerobic activities, be sure to do your joint warm-ups and a dynamic warm-up before beginning this activity. Stay within your heart rate zone and do not exceed your maximum zone. Wear protective gear if possible. There are other safety considerations in this sport. Be certain you are aware of them and adhere to them.

- Martial Arts. Take breaks as necessary to stay within your target heart rate zone. Remember that you won't be able to talk much but you won't be just gasping for air. If you find that you are, slow down. Although this is a sport that can be started at any age, it is best learned under the guidance of a professional. Seek certified guidance, preferably with a highly recommended gym or studio. Strictly follow your instructor's advice.

- Boxing. Take breaks as necessary to stay within your target heart rate zone. Remember that you won't be able to talk much, but you won't be just gasping for air. Follow your coach's directions to the letter. His vast knowledge is invaluable to you.

- Trampoline. Take breaks as necessary to stay within your target heart rate zone. Remember that you won't be able to talk much, but you won't be just gasping for air. If you find that you are, slow down.

- Rowing. Take breaks as necessary to stay within your target heart rate zone. Remember that you won't be able to talk much, but you won't be just gasping for air. If you find that you are, slow down. As with all cardio/aerobic activities, begin with a joint warm-up as well as a dynamic warm-up such as jumping jacks, squats, and burpees. These will get your blood flowing to warm your muscles, your heartbeat slightly elevated, and you keep your breathing up.

- Stair Climbing. Take breaks as necessary to stay within your target heart rate zone. Remember that you won't be able to talk much, but you won't be just gasping for air. If you find that you are, slow down. Drink plenty of fluids, and be certain you are wearing footgear that will prevent any slips. In addition to your joint warm-ups, a good dynamic warm-up should include squats that strengthen the knee muscles to prepare them for the work ahead.

Further Increasing Your Capacity

o   As with the Beginning Cardio/Aerobics Workout, you will eventually become so fit that you will no longer find this Advanced Cardio/Aerobics Workout a challenge, or you find you easily stay in the low end of your target heart rate zone. That's when you know it's time to up your game and move into athlete level cardio/aerobics workouts.

Athlete Level Cardio/Aerobics

Many of the workouts that are in the Advanced Cardio/Aerobics Workout can be moved into the Athlete Level Cardio/Aerobics category simply by playing at a higher intensity. Did you pick basketball? Play one-on-one with someone who is nearly as good or even better than you. Boxing or Martial Arts? Try competing. You will have to spar more often to prepare for competition, and you will have to choose better opponents. You will also have to work at maximum capacity if you hope to win.

Strength training within an aerobic capacity is also excellent for athlete level cardio/aerobics. Check out Chapter 3: Strength Training>Cardio/Aerobics Strength Training Suggested Workouts.

Cool Down

The cool down allows your heart rate and blood pressure to slowly return to normal. It also allows your muscles to cool slowly, thus preventing injury. Stretching after a workout can reduce the buildup of lactic acid, preventing muscle cramps and stiffness.

- Walk for about 5 minutes until your heart gets below 120 beats per minute.
- Stretch
    - Hold each stretch for at least 20 seconds.
    - Breathe in, and while you're doing this, hold the stretch.
    - Lengthen the stretch or further it as you exhale.
    - Here are some sample stretches to try:
        - Toe touch stretch: with legs spread, bend over and let your upper body weight stretch your hands to the ground. Once your back is comfortably relaxed in this position, rotate towards your right foot without swiveling your hips. Keep your hips parallel to the ground and only move your arms. You will feel the stretch at the back of your thighs as well as the back of your arms. Hold.
    - Gently move your arms to the other side. Hold.
        - Lunge: Stand with feet hip-width apart. Bend your left knee, leaning and stretching towards the left. That way, your inner right thigh is stretched. Your hips will thrust back somewhat. Hold for 20 seconds or more. Push back up to center. Repeat to the right.
        - Hip flexor stretch: From the lunge position, turn towards either leg. Bend the forward leg while pressing down and forward with the hips and stretching out on the toes of the back foot. The stretch is in the hip of the back-stretching leg. Tilt yourself back in the calf stretch below before switching legs.
        - Calf Stretch: Standing, put one foot forward. Stretch down to toes. Pull toes towards your body until you feel a gentle stretch in your calf. You can also wrap a towel around your foot and pull both sides of the towel towards your face to produce this stretch. Hold for twenty seconds. Switch sides. Alternately, this can be

done seated. Incorporate this with the hip flexor stretch above by doing first the hip flexor and then the calf stretch on one side, then moving to the other side to do both stretches.

- Toe touches: You did a variation of these in your warm-up. This time, stand with your feet together. Let your bodyweight pull your upper body towards your toes. Hang for 20 seconds or longer. With each exhale, allow your upper body to stretch closer to your toes. Relax your entire back from your neck along the length of your spine over your buttocks down the back of your thighs. With each exhale, allow your body weight to stretch your muscles further. Roll up very slowly and that way, you don't get dizzy.

- Side stretch: With feet hip-width apart and arms out like a windmill, bend to the side. One arm tilts down towards your leg, while the other stays parallel, reaching for the sky. Only your torso moves. Reach as far down your leg as you can and hold this pose. Pivot at the waist to make this a twisting side stretch by taking your hand to the opposite ankle. After a hold on that stretch, return to the starting leg. Hold again. Rise up to the start position. Repeat on the opposite side.

- Overhead arm stretch: This is simple. You probably do this every morning. Grasp your hands together, reach overhead. Stretch. Hold for 20 seconds. Add to this beautiful stretch by leaning slightly to one side, hold, lean to the other side, hold. You're done.

- A simple yoga sun salutation is an excellent cool down stretch:
  - Start standing feet together (Mountain Pose).

- Join your palms over your head (Raised Arms Pose), lean slightly back.
- Bend forward at the waist taking your hands together to the floor. (Forward Bend Uttanasana)
- Walk your hands forward, moving up on your toes. Press your head between your hands. (Downward-Facing Dog). This provides a lovely stretch between your shoulder blades, up over your back, and down your hamstrings. Press your heels into the ground gently so that you don't tear your Achilles tendon.
- Inhale as you move forward into Planking Pose. This is the typical push up pose. Round your shoulders out so that you do not collapse between your shoulder blades. Suck your belly button towards your backbone. Tuck your pelvis and firm your thighs.
- Push back slightly and scoop your chest as low to the ground as possible as you slip up like a snake into the Cobra Pose. Do not let your chest touch the ground until you have scooped all the way through your hands. Now control your descent to the ground. Your whole body will be low to the ground.
- Push up into the Upward Facing Dog. Your body is supported on your hands and toes. Keep a tight torso.
- Push back, keeping your hands in the same spot on the floor, bending at the knees, sitting on your heels. You are now in Child's Pose.

Hold this pose that stretches your back from hamstrings through to your neck.

o Move up onto all fours. Now, arch your back. Suck in your belly. Push yourself the Cat Pose.

o Reverse the arch so your head is up and your belly is down. This is the Cow Pose. Repeat these two moves (Cat and Cow) slowly several times.

o Take one arm and Thread the Needle by thrusting between your other arm and body bring your active arm's shoulder to the ground. Your body will twist, stretching your back and waist. Hold on an exhale. Take a deep breath. Return to all fours. Thread the opposite Needle. Return to all fours.

o Sit back in Child's Pose.

o Rise up to Downward-Facing Dog

o Walk fingers back towards toes. Slowly roll up one vertebra at a time until you are back at Mountain Pose.

o Lift your arms overhead with palms together to Raised Arms Pose.

o Bring arms back to chest with hands still pressed together to Prayer Pose. Breath deep and quiet.

Keeping Up Your Interest

Variety is the key to keeping up your interest. Today you walked outside for your workout. Tomorrow, try dancing to your favorite tunes. The next day, when it rains, use a treadmill. The day after that, do calisthenics. Don't forget that each week will be broken up with your two to three days of strength training. These can be done together or interspersed during your week.

Or maybe you're not bored so easily, and you can do one exercise for a week or even two weeks before you feel the slightest bit bored. But if you have any feelings of wanting to stop working out, first try switching up your routine to put a little excitement back into your workout. You might even try something you've never done before – like mountain biking. Or spin class. Or ballroom dancing.

Perhaps you only need to change your venue to keep your interest. For the first half of the week, do all you exercise indoors. For the second half of the week, make sure every workout is outside.

Tips and Tricks to Fit Cardio/Aerobics Time in When You're Under Time Tension

The higher your athletic ability, the quicker your workout can be and still meet the American Heart Association Guidelines for Fitness. You have to workout 150 minutes per week if you're on the beginner level (37 ½ minutes four days per week plus two strength training days). You can break this down to two 18 ¾ minutes twice a day.

Do you need to break it down further? How about four 10 minute sessions per day? You can do that with quick calisthenics workouts easily. Just take the dog out for a fast walk or if your dog runs around off-leash, take the time while he's sniffing to do some fast squats, trunk twists, lunges, and knee lifts until his outdoor time is up. That should be about ten minutes. It's a quick, useful, and impactful workout. And you've squeezed it into doggy poop time. Good for you!

Try jumping rope with a weighted rope. Because jump rope is such an intense workout, you can fit a quick workout in with less time than a run. If you add the benefit of a weighted rope, you are also adding some strength training benefits that create an even more intense workout. You can cut your workout from 18 ¾ minutes down to 12 minutes.

Strength training is one of the easiest workouts to squeeze in quickly because you can do it anywhere. Truthfully. Your body is your weight. So anywhere you are, you have resistance to strength train against. See more information in Chapter 3: Strength Training>Bodyweight Resistance.

Combine your aerobics workout with strength training, and you've done two workouts at once. That can give you an extra day off. But don't take more than two days a week off. You need the consistency of at least five days of workout/week.

Now let me share a little secret with you. The quickest aerobic/strength training workout you can do is just three little moves that cover your whole body. Yep. Bench press, deadlift, and squat. Or substitute thrusters for the deadlift. Do this one after the other in the aerobic capacity, and you can do a full-body workout in no time. You've got time for that! Read on.

CHAPTER 3: STRENGTH TRAINING

One of the difficulties of aging is that you lose muscle mass after age thirty, and you have lower testosterone after age 40. You need strength training to maintain and increase muscle mass and boost your testosterone. Did you know it could do that? That's why it's so essential to men – especially those over 50, like you.

Warm-Up

As with our cardio/aerobics workouts, we want to warm-up our joints first. See Chapter 2: Cardio/Aerobics>Warm-Up>Joint Warm-Up. Get the synovial fluid flowing.

Form Is Everything

Next, we need a dynamic warm-up. Since dynamic warm-ups should be geared toward the exercise you are about to do, we want the dynamic warm-up we do right now to be geared toward strength training.

Since *Form is Everything,* we're going to perform each of these warm-up moves with the best form possible. Think of it as training for the weight moves as we use them in our strength training routines. Pick several of the moves below to warm-up for about five minutes before you begin your strength training workout.

- **Jumping Jacks**: This is just a warm-up and about fifteen reps are enough.
- **Running in the Same Place** without moving for one minute.
- **Bodyweight Squats**: This should be a no-brainer. Our bodies are designed to squat. Before the chair, it's what we did. A simple bodyweight squat uses almost every muscle in your core (this is so important) and your lower body. Conquer

these. In strength training, this is one of the major moves because, combined with thrusters or deadlifts and bench press, these three moves cover your whole body. You can have the best full-body workout available in no time flat with just three moves. Your form is *everything*. So get it right *now*.

o   Start with feet just slightly more than hip-width apart.

o   Point your toes slightly outward.

o   Focus your eyes on a spot straight in front of you and keep your eyes focused there throughout the move.

o   Put your arms straight out, parallel to the ground, chest up, spine neutral. Keep your chest up.

o   Keep your weight on the balls of your feet and your heels. There is no weight on your toes.

o   Keep your core tight as it is supporting you through this move.

o   Break at your hip and sit into your butt, pushing your hips backward as though they are reaching for a chair. Think about sitting, not about bending your knees.

o   Focus on pushing your knees out but not wider than your feet. Do not let them move towards each other.

o   Squat until your hip joints are lower than your knees. That's the bottom of the move.

o   Now think of driving your heels into the ground to reverse the move as you squeeze your butt and press your knees outward to rise back up.

o   Repeat this move until it is perfect and comfortable. Only then will you be ready to add weight.

o   For the warm-up Bodyweight Squats, repeat in perfect form 10-15 times.

o   **Hip Extensions**: Lie on your back. Bend knees placing feet flat on the ground. Thrust hips towards the sky, tucking hips upwards. Hold. Lower to ground.

o   **Hip Rotations**: Stand with arms out to the sides. Lift leg to the front at hip height with the knee bent. Rotate to one side and lower to the ground. Lift and rotate to front. Repeat five times on each leg.

- o **Forward Leg Swings**: Stand with one hand holding a bar or wall or something for support. Swing outside leg forward and backward. Swing with some control and not higher than hip. Too much swing risks injury. Aim to follow these guidelines.
- o **Side Leg Swings**: Hold bar or wall in front of you. Swing leg across the body and out to the side. As with forward leg swings, swing with some control and not higher than hip. Too much swing risks injury and therefore, be sure to follow these guidelines.
- o **Push Up**: Start in the planking pose. Think of squeezing a walnut between your shoulder blades. Start at an incline. You can do these against a door with just a slight incline, then progress to a steeper and steeper incline until your parallel to the floor. The closer to parallel you go, the harder the push up becomes. Lower your body until your chest touches the ground. Push all the way back up. Be sure your whole body is tight as you perform this move and that you remain in the planking pose, without letting your butt pop up.

There are many push up variations. See Bodyweight Resistance Sample Body Weight Resistance Routines for more examples. For warm-up purposes, a simple push up is fine.

- o **Mountain Climbers:** This is a great last-move for your warm-up because it will amp up your body temperature and really get the blood flowing through your muscles so that they are primed and ready for a good strength training workout. Here we go.
- o In the planking position, same as for the push ups you just did, your hands are shoulder-width apart, your back is flat, your

39

abs are tight, and your weight is evenly distributed between your hands, and toes.

- o Bring one knee towards your elbow, touching your toe beneath your chest.
- o Bounce back, switching feet under you. Your hands remain stable as your feet switch back and forth, alternately touching beneath your chest.

Bodyweight Resistance

The Advantages of Body Resistance

Strength training is essential to your workout regime because it helps you build and maintain muscle that you naturally lose to aging. We already know that. The advantage of bodyweight resistance, as opposed to weight machines, free weights, or even resistance bands, is that you always have your bodyweight with you. There is nowhere that you can't perform bodyweight resistance strength training. You never have an excuse. Have a few minutes while you're waiting for your wife to come out from a visit with a friend? Great – bodyweight squats. Commercials are running, and you haven't put in today's workout? No problem – drop and give me 20 – bodyweight resistance push ups, that is. Or pyramid push ups for a little extra shoulder definition. Or gecko crawls across the living room for a little more of an aerobic workout.

There is simply no end to what bodyweight resistance workouts can do for you and your body.

Sample Body Weight Resistance Exercises

- o **Six Inch Hold:** Lie on your back, legs straight, arms at your side with hands just under your butt. Raise your left leg six inches or so off the matt. Pull belly to your spine to keep low back from lifting off the matt. Hold for 30 seconds to a minute.

- o **Leg Lift:** Same position as for six-inch hold. Again, the belly is pulled towards the spine. Lift legs towards the ceiling, keeping your knees straight. Slowly lower back towards flower pushing low back into the ground bring legs to just an inch off the floor. Use abdominal strength, not momentum, to lift legs. Repeat.
- o **Bicycle Crunch:** Still in the same position as for leg lifts with your belly pulled towards your spine for good abdominal support. Pull knee to opposite elbow over abdomen while the other leg remains straight. Reverse by straightening the bent knee and tucking your opposite knee to your elbow. Continue to reverse rapidly but with good form for a count of 10-20 reps.
- o **Windshield Wiper – Beware of your back in this move.** Move slowly and with strong abdominal support. On your back, brace your arms straight out in a "T" from your body. Raise legs towards the ceiling parallel to your torso. Lower legs as far to the side as possible without lifting shoulders. With the strength of your abdomen, move them to the other side and lower as close to the floor as possible, again without lifting your shoulders. Alternate from side to side with determined control.
- o **Superman:** Lie face down. Extend hands to allow the body to be stretched in a long line from feet to fingers. Lift arms, chest, and legs off the floor all at once as though you are like Superman, flying in the sky. Contract your body while relaxing your shoulders and neck. Hold. Relax. Repeat.
- o **Swimmer:** This is the same move as the superman, only this time, when you lift your arms and legs into the air, you are going to perform a swimming motion by kicking the opposite leg while lifting the opposing arm, then switching leg and arm. Continue alternating for 30 to 60 seconds. Rest. Repeat. This is an awesome core workout.
- o Push Up Variations

41

- Crawl out to push up: Start in the basic planking position. Do a push up when you come up from the floor, crawl hands back towards feet while pushing bottom into the air until hands and feet are together. Stand up. Lower your hands to the floor. Walk hands out until you are once again in the planking pose. Repeat.
- Planking March: Start in basic planking position, remembering to keep your core tight with belly pulled in to spine. Spread feet wider than usual for stability. Bend one elbow lowering forearm to the floor. Lower your other forearm to the floor. Extend the first arm, extend the second arm returning you to planking position. Keep your body as still and firm as possible during this move. Repeat.
- Gecko Crawl, also called "Walking Gecko Push up": Start with a regular push up. But when you come up, you bring one leg forward and the opposite leg forward as you go down into a deep push up. Reverse on the other side. Go forward about five steps, then back for the same number. Only do as many as you can in good form.
- Bird Dog: On hands and knees, bring bent elbow to bent knee beneath body while maintaining a flat back. Extend to straight out. Repeat for a count of 10. Switch sides.
- Donkey Kick: On your hands and knees, keep your leg bent at a 90° angle. Tuck your chin slightly. Engage your lower abdominals to prevent your spine from rounding. Lift your right knee slowly up and towards the ceiling. Raise to the point before your back starts to arch or your hips begin to rotate. Lower back down and repeat. Do 8 – 10 reps. Switch legs. This exercise targets your glutes while stretching your hip in the opposite direction of the way we sit. If you have a desk job, this exercise works the kinks back out from all that sitting. It helps improve posture and prevent spine and hip injuries.

o **Burpee:** Stand with feet hip-width apart. Drop hands to the ground. Thrust feet out. Drop chest to the ground. Quickly jump feet back to hands. Jump up and thrust hands to the sky. Drop hands to sides. Repeat. You're burpin'.

o **Triceps Dip:** Sit on a chair bench, or box with your feet together and a good distance out. Put your hands on the edge of the seat. Lift and slide your hips off the seat. Bend your elbows to lower yourself towards the floor. Push up until elbows are straight. Dip down to the ground. Repeat.

These are just a few of the many bodyweight resistance strength training exercises you can do. You can find more on the internet or in books devoted to strength training.

Let's look at some bodyweight resistance moves for cardio/aerobic work.

Cardio/Aerobic Bodyweight Resistance suggested workout for Beginner Level Work out

o **Burpees:** Burpees will always be one of my favorite bodyweight resistance work out moves. It's great, no matter what your fitness level is. For the beginner, you are going to slow this move down so that you stay within your target heartbeat range. When you start to get winded and pass that range, take a break and walk in circles.

o Here's a little parenting/grandparenting trick. If you have a child/grandchild that's getting a little overly excited, teach them to do a burpee. Whenever you need to get the energy out of them quickly, have them demonstrate good burpees to you. Just ask, "show me how you do a burpee." Then have them show you again. And again. And again. Until you see that they are pretty worn out. This is actually a pretty fun exercise to do for a little kid – even for us bigger kids. And it is an excellent full-body workout. So while you are wearing out your kiddo, you are also doing them a good turn because you are giving them the benefit of bodywork and heart work.

o Here's how you do it: Stand with feet hip-width apart. Drop hands to the ground. Thrust feet out. Drop chest to the ground. Quickly jump feet back to hands. Jump up and thrust hands to the sky. Drop hands to sides. Repeat. You're burpin'.

o **Kang Squat:** You've perfected your squat technique at the beginning of this chapter. Here's a high-intensity variation to put you in cardio/aerobic workout mode.

o In your perfect squat position, place your hands behind your head. Hing at your hips and bend, that way, your upper body is parallel with the ground. Perform your squat. Push your heels through the ground to reverse the movement returning the body parallel to the ground position, and then lift the body upright to a stand. Repeat. Control your movement, especially the bending over at the waist, as this can throw off your balance.

o **Lateral Squat Walk:** In a perfect squat position, lower slightly. Maintaining a half-squat position, step to the right. Step to the right again. Step left, step left. Be sure to maintain the half-squat position throughout the movement. Repeat.

o **Staggered-Stance Deadlift**: Stand with feet slightly apart, and well-balanced. Take a slight step back to balance on the left foot. Brace left hand over the right wrist. With your weight on the front (right) leg, bend knees while pushing hips back until hamstring stretches, keeping torso parallel to the floor. Reach your fingertips towards the right foot in front of the shin. Keep back flat. Return to standing. Repeat about ten times. Switch legs. Repeat.

o **Alternating See-Saw Lunge:** This requires a tight core throughout. Step forward into a lunge, curling the opposite arm up and touching the back knee to the ground. Instead of coming back to standing, swing the forward leg back and down to kneeling until you are now in a lunge on the opposite leg while curling the opposite arm up. Return to standing. That is one full rep. Repeat. Switch sides.

o **Inch Worm:** If you're familiar with yoga, this is what you do to get to downward-facing dog, except with feet farther apart and you take it all the way to planking position. If you're not into yoga, stand with feet hip-width apart, bend to place your hands on the floor in front of you, and begin walking them out alternately away from you until you are stretched out onto your toes, and your hands are under your shoulders in the planking position. Now walk your hands back to your feet and roll up to standing, lifting your hands high overhead. *Make it harder: **Inch Worm Planking:*** Same move but this time, when you get down to the planking position, add a push up before walking your hands back to your feet.

o **Mountain Climber Twist**: Start in basic planking position. Bring one knee under your body towards the opposite elbow. As you extend it back to its place, bring the other knee to the opposite elbow. The faster you go, the higher the cardio. Just be sure to keep your core tight and your movements precise. No sloppy flopping around here.

o **Planking Jack:** You're already in the planking position. Keeping your core tight, you're now going to do a jumping jack move with your feet. Jump them apart, then together as quickly as possible while keeping your hips level. Repeat this move. The faster you go, the more aerobic it is. Just be certain you maintain good plank form with a tight core.

o **Plank-to-Knee Tap:** Still in your tight-core planking position, this time you're going to lift your body at the hips into the air so you can touch one hand to the opposite knee, then return to the planking before lifting to touch the other hand to opposite knee. Continue to switch hands to knees as quickly as possible. *Make it harder: **Corkscrew:*** Same move,

45

only this time you will kick your toe all the way to the side when you cross your leg under your body, and you will reach your hand out to touch it. Maintain a tight core throughout.

o **Triceps Push up with Mountain Climber:** Mountain climber, mountain climber, then stop in the planking position, lower yourself to your elbows (triceps push up), lift yourself back up. Repeat. If this move is a tad too difficult, lower one elbow at a time. Either way, you will quickly get into a cardio/aerobic state.

o **Sprinter Sit-Up:** This is a difficult move, and you will want to perform a few, rest by grasping legs to chest and rocking, then perform a few more and repeat the resting motion. Start in a sit-up position. Extend on the leg and bring the opposite knee, and elbow together across the body. Keeping a tight core, switch your knees and elbow. Continue switching in a steady motion. Up the difficulty by increasing the speed.

o **Squat Jump:** Do a perfect squat – you are going to be so good at these – with your hands behind your head. When you get to the bottom, give yourself an enormous burst through your heels while pushing your arms down for momentum to launch yourself into the air. Land lightly on your toes to drop back into that perfect squat and start all over again.

o **Box Step:** This is a little like stair climbing. You are going to use a box, a bench, or anything that is mid calf height (to start – move higher as you become more fit). Stand with feet shoulder-width apart. Step up with one foot, then the other. Step back down with the starting foot and then the other. Now, reverse the direction of your feet for the next step.

o **Bear Crawl:** Of the crawling exercises, this is one of the easiest. It is a full-body exercise. You can start on all fours, but the proper position is something more, like a cross between all fours and downward-facing dog. You need to be in a comfortable, hands and toes pose that allows you the most agility. Your hips will be higher than your shoulders. You will be on your toes as though you are launching yourself out of sprinter's blocks. Moving as lightly as possible, cover as much ground as possible as quickly as possible, moving forward on hands and toes. You are a grizzly rushing towards its prey. You are a huge, swift, lumbering animal.

o **Crab Walk:** Flip over to your back. Lift your body on your hands and feet, thrusting your hips into the air and maintaining a tight core. Walk forwards and backward.

o **Superman:** This is as good for your core as a sit-up. Laying on your belly, tighten your core, and lift both arms and both legs off the ground at the same time. Hold. *Variation: Swim:* Kick arms and legs. *Roll:* Keeping your core very tight, roll over onto your back. You will have to arch your arms and legs upwards as you move onto your back. Continue to roll, reversing arms and legs as you move from belly to back. This is an excellent full-body workout that tightens your core in the way that sit-ups do but works your entire abdomen instead of just a small part of it. When you string all three of these exercises together, you turn this move into a cardio/aerobic exercise.

Cardio/Aerobic Bodyweight Resistance suggested workout for Advanced Level Workouts

o **Squat Lunge**: Start in your perfect squat position with your hands clasped in front of your chest. Squat. Follow with a step forward into a lunge. Lower into a lunge and step back. Lower to squat. Step the other leg forward to a lunge. Lower to lunge. Rise and step back. Repeat.

o **Side to Side Squat Jump:** In your perfect squat position, lower into half a squat. Swing your arms forward and use the moment to help you jump to the right landing in a squat. Swing and jump back to the start. That's one rep. Repeat.

47

- Burpee Jump Ups: Stand with feet hip-width apart. Drop hands to the ground. Thrust feet out. Drop chest to the ground. Quickly jump feet back to hands. Jump up and burst into the air jumping off of the ground. Repeat.

- Sumo Squat Jack – When you go down into your squat, you are going to cross your arms in front of your chest. Push back up with energy into the closed position of a jumping jack with your feet together and your hands together over your head. Do the second half of the jumping jack landing with your feet spread in a squat and your hands crossed over your chest in the squat position you started in. Repeat energetically.

- Spiderman Lunge and Squat – Start in your squat position with hands in a prayer position in front of you. Place hands on the ground just in front of your legs. Lunge back to the planking pose. Hold for only a moment. Bring legs forward to starting position one at a time (ala spiderman). Bring hands back to prayer position. Repeat. The faster you do this, the more aerobic it becomes.

- Skaters: With feet hip-width apart, you are going to jump from one foot to the other, bringing the lifted foot behind as your opposite hand swing to the front across the body to help maintain balance. Sweep back to the other side, landing on the opposite foot. This is a high cardio/aerobic move because both your feet and arms are vigorously moving.

- Long Jump with Jog-Back: Jog back four or five steps and you will be able to calculate this better after you jump forward with both feet as far as you can while landing solidly on both feet. How far you jumped forward is about as far as you want to jog back. Repeat.

- Dive Bomber Push up: If you do yoga, this is downward-facing dog to upward facing dog. Start with your feet slightly apart, bend at the waist and place your hands on the floor far enough in front of you that your body forms a nice triangle and you are slightly on your toes. Bend your arms as you slide your chin down along the ground and through your hands up into the air until your hips graze the floor, and your chin continues up into the air until you are looking up with your hips and legs on the ground like a dive bomber. Reverse the movement rotating your head down as you lift your hips backward and back to the lifted hip position.

o **Runner's Skip:** Drop to a low lunge with back leg extended rather than dropped to a knee and hand on that side touching the ground. Jump up, lifting the extended leg's knee to chest height. Drop back down as quickly as possible while maintaining good form. Repeat about five times before switching sides.

o **Flutter Kicks:** Lie on your back, keeping a tight core. Put hands on the ground at your sides or under your low back. Lift both feet a few inches off the ground and kick feet up and down several inches, fluttering them. This should not cause low back pain. If it does, discontinue. *Alternate*: Rather than fluttering up and down, cross feet over and under.

o **Box Jump:** You are going to use a box, a bench, or anything that is mid calf height (to start – move higher as you become more fit). Stand with feet shoulder-width apart. Bend knees and swing arms back. Jump lightly up onto the box. Step back down one foot at a time. Repeat, stepping down with the opposite foot leading.

o **Donkey Kick:** Start in planking position with a nice tight core. Kick bent feet into the air at the same time to slightly higher than butt while coming somewhat forward on arms. Land lightly on toes and repeat.

o **Lateral Jump:** Do this over a low bench. With the bench to your right, shift your weight to your left foot. Jump over the bench leading with your right foot. Land on your right foot.

Jump back over the bench leading with your left foot. Land on your left foot. Repeat.

o **Push up Variations:** There are lots of push up variations, all of which can quickly work you into a cardio/aerobic state. Be sure to remain aware of your target heart rate zone and your maximum heart rate while doing these. Additionally, since each variation works different muscles, be aware of what part of your body aches the next day. If you have *sharp* pain in your neck, back or shoulders immediately following a particular push up or the next day, be certain that you used proper form. If you did, and you still have that pain, discontinue that particular push up.

Remember that the greater your angle, the less effort your push up will require.

o Here are some push up Variations to try:

o **Plyometric push up:** This is a jumping push up. Do a traditional push up, but on the way up, explode upwards so that you come off the ground. To see some absolutely beautiful examples of plyometric push ups please view the introduction of this video:

https://www.youtube.com/watch ?v=5Ssun8IqkD4

o **Drop push ups:** Do this push up on benches or steps or rings or pretty much anything you can lower your body between. Again, the greater the angle of your body, the less effort the move will require. The closer to parallel to the ground, the greater your effort. Place your hands on the benches or rings with your body in the planking position. Next, lower your body between them by bending your elbows and thrusting your chest between them. If you are parallel to the ground, you may lower until your chest touches the ground. Push back up to the planking position. Repeat.

- Spiderman Push ups: This is one of my favorites. Not only is it a great exercise that can build cardio/aerobics, but it also looks really cool. Want to get a kid exercising? Teach 'em to do Spiderman push ups. Then teach them to *move* while doing it. Here's how to do it:
- From the planking position, lift knee to elbow as you lower, turning your head towards that side.
- Lift yourself back to the planking position.
- Lower to other side turning head to that side while lifting that knee to elbow.
- Keep your toes relaxed throughout.
- Walking Gecko Push up: Take spidey to the next level.
- Start in the planking position.
- Lower to regular push up.
- Step arm and opposite foot forward as you rise. You will look like spiderman or a gecko as the knee is bent.
- Lower to the bent knee, bent arm position, then lift to the opposite bent knee and arm moving forward.
- Move forward, doing the move several steps. Then backward, doing several steps.
- *Variation Chameleon*: Lift high between each forward move, then lift again, raising non-weight bearing arm and leg into the air and lower and lift before moving forward onto the opposite side.
- Pseudo Planche Push Up: To do this push up, you will put your hands closer to your waist. The More forward you lean, the more difficult it becomes. In other words, the closer your hands are to your waist, the more bodyweight you are lifting. Protract the scapula for clean execution. Now lower and lift as for a normal push up.
- Sphinx Push ups: To focus on the triceps when you perform this move. In a standard planking position, bring your hands closer together under your face. Lower by bending your

elbows until you are resting on your forearms. Vary the intensity by moving forward and backward on the arms. Bend knees to the ground to decrease intensity.

- o **Archer Push ups**: Do these to prepare yourself for the one-arm push up. Simply move your body further and further over one arm as you do your push up. Do this until you can do them so far to the side that you are using only a few fingers of the outstretched arm. Now you're ready to attempt a one-arm push up.

- o **Pike push ups:** Use the downward-facing dog position (On your toes, bent to a triangle, resting on your hands), lower your head through your arms down to the ground. Slide back up, lifting your head up and between your arms. This is a straight move with no arching.

- o **Back bridge push up**: This increases mobility in the shoulders. Do not do this one if you have lower back issues. To make it easier, you can keep your head on the ground. Starting on your back, you will balance on your feet or the balls of your feet, and your hands will be flat next to your ears. Press up into a bridge. Holding this position, lower till your shoulders touch the ground, then lift yourself back up. *Variation to increase intensity:* Lift one leg while performing the movement.

Cardio/Aerobic Bodyweight Resistance suggested workout for Athletic Level Workouts

- o **Push up Variations:** There are lots of push up variations all of which can quickly work you into a cardio/aerobic state. Be sure to remain aware of your target heart rate zone and your maximum heart rate while doing these. Additionally, since each variation works different muscles, be aware of what part of your body aches the next day. If you have *sharp* pain in your neck, back or shoulders immediately following a particular push up, or the next day, be certain that you used proper form. If you did, and you still have that pain, discontinue that particular push up.

o Remember that the greater your angle, the less effort your push up will require.

o Here are some push up Variations to try:

o **Walking Gecko Push up:** Take spidey to the next level.

o Start in the planking position.

o Lower to regular push up.

o Step arm and opposite foot forward as you rise. You will look like spiderman or a gecko as the knee is bent.

o Lower to the bent knee, bent arm position, then lift to the opposite bent knee and arm moving forward.

o Move forward with this motion for several steps. Then step backward several steps.

o *Variation Chameleon*: Lift high between each forward move then left again, raising your non-weight bearing arm and leg into the air and lower and lift before moving forward onto the opposite side.

o **Pseudo Planche Push Up:** To do this push- p, you will put your hands closer to your waist. The More forward you lean, the more difficult it becomes. In other words, the closer your hands are to your waist, the more bodyweight you are lifting. Protract the scapula for clean execution. Now lower and lift as for a normal push up.

o **Tuck Planche:** Do this between two push up bars. Place your hands on the bars that should be shoulder-width apart. Tuck your body up between your arms until you are supporting yourself. Lower your body between your arms and down past your hands till you're almost touching the ground. Press back up. Repeat.

o **Planche Push Up:** For those of you who are really advanced and have practiced the pseudo planche push up, moving your hands closer and closer to your waist, you are ready to perform planche push ups. In this push up, your hands are at your waist, with your fingers facing out. Lean forward on your arms with your butt in the air, almost as though you were going to perform a pyramid push up. This will help you to lift your feet off the ground when your body balances between your elbows. Press up. Lower down. Your body remains extended and in the air. Repeat.

o **One-arm push ups:** High intensity with core stability comes from this exercise. Your body will maintain a strong core with no sagging through your hips. Do Archer Push ups to prepare for these. Put one arm behind your back, lower your body to the flower and push back up. Simple, huh?

o **Back bridge push up**: This increases mobility in the shoulders. Do not do this one if you have lower back issues. To make it easier, you can keep your head on the ground. Starting on your back, you will balance on your feet or the balls of your feet, and your hands will be flat next to your ears. Press up into a bridge. Holding this position, lower till your shoulders touch the ground, then lift yourself back up. *Variation to increase intensity:* Lift one leg while performing the movement.

o **The Planking Jack:** Start in the planking position as though you were about to do a push up. Jump your feet apart, landing on your toes, and then quickly jumping them back together. Keep your core tight and firm. Your shoulders are going to burn. Land lightly. Your abs will work hard. Keep it up for a full minute. Rest 30 seconds. Repeat.

o **Body Saw:** Rest your elbows on a padded surface, put your body in the planking position with your feet on a slippery surface, as you will need to slide your feet back and forth. With a very firm core, slide your feet out, sawing your body back away from your body and extending your arms back so that your arms are stretched, and your body is in a nearly straight line from arms to feet. Pull back in.

- o **Crab Planking Walk:** In the planking position, walk leg and arm on the same side a small step out. Step the other side in the same direction. You will be 'crab crawling' to the side. Take a few steps in one direction. Stop. Do a full push up. Crawl in the opposite direction. Do a full push up. Repeat.

- o **Side Planking Crunch:** From a strong planking position, pivot your whole body to one side so that you are balanced on the outside of your bottom foot and the elbow of your bottom arm. Pull your top elbow to your knee, crunching your side. Extend. That's one rep. Repeat as many times as you can in one minute, then turn to the other side and do the same.

- o **Shadow Box:** Jab and punch with your arms keeping your elbows tucked tight to your body, twisting at the waist. Pivot on your feet, shuffling, bouncing, keeping continuous motion going, switching which foot is in front, double stepping, etc. Keep movement up as quickly as possible for one solid minute before resting for 30 seconds.

Weight Machines

Proper form prevents any kind of injury from taking place

Most of the time, if you are working on weight machines, you will be working at a gym. Most gyms offer you a free introduction to the machines when you sign up. This introduction usually includes adjusting the machines to your body size and figuring out your initial starting weight. Do not be afraid to adjust these after your initial introduction.

Chances are, you were moved through this process fairly rapidly. Your instructor may not have taken the proper time to adjust everything perfectly. If you feel uncomfortable with a move, like your muscle is not being fully extended or until your body slumps a little bit, feel free to extend or lower the seat to get the proper positioning. Ask for assistance if you need it.

The advantage of weight machines is that they guide you through the proper motion. It is difficult to use a weight machine with poor form. With few exceptions, arching your back is poor form. If you are doing lat pull-downs or rowing, you *do* need to arch your back. Otherwise, your back should remain straight and flat. In all other moves, the machine itself leads you through proper motion.

If you feel really sore, you have lifted too much weight. Cut back. You should never feel more than mildly sore. That soreness is why people stop lifting weights or working out at all. Weight lifting is essential to good overall health, especially as you age and naturally lose muscle. For men, this is especially important since losing muscle also contributes to losing testosterone. When you lose testosterone, you become more flabby, looking more and more feminine rather than having the muscle tone that is attributed to a masculine physique.

Proper Weight

The proper weight is one you can lift about ten times, feeling that the last two or three are difficult, but not impossible.

Adding Weight

When and How

When you can whip out ten repetitions with no effort, you need more weight. Add five pounds. If that is still very little effort, continue to add five pounds until you feel moderate effort throughout and quite a bit of effort on the last two or three repetitions – but not as though it's nearly impossible.

How to know if you've added too Much

If you feel seriously strained when you lift a weight, if you cannot make ten repetitions, if you are seriously sore the next day, you have done too much weight. Cut back. Follow the guidelines above to know when and how to add weight. Ten repetitions is a good number of reps to shoot for. Add weight if you can easily do more reps. Cut back on weight if you can only do eight reps.

Sample Weight Machine Workout

These are the eight machines you should use – skip the rest and use bodyweight resistance or free weights instead.

Lat Pull-Down: This machine works the broadest muscle of your back as well as your shoulders. If you're going to do pull-ups (bodyweight resistance), start with lat pull-downs to work your way into the strength to do them. Beginners: use an under grasp with your palms facing you for an easier move that uses more biceps. For more challenge, bring your hands closer together or spread them apart in a V-shape.

Pull-up/Dip Machine: This machine helps you use proper form once you're ready to move from Lat Pull-downs to Pull-ups. Dips are every bit as hard as pull-ups. Because this machine reduces the percentage of your bodyweight that you're actually lifting, it allows you to maintain good form while building strength in your upper body. You can also perform triceps dips on this machine.

Hanging Leg Raise: This works your core and your hip flexors. Prop your forearms on the machine and lift your legs in a slow and controlled motion. Legs can be lifted straight out or bent up to the chest, or pulled bent to either side.

Seated Row Machine: This is a total body, cardio machine.

Chest Press: For your chest, biceps, and triceps, this machine gives you a motion very much like a push up. Relax your legs but keep your core engaged as you thrust with your arms and rock back with this move. Remember that one of the advantages of weight machines is that they guide your form, thus preventing injury.

Seated Leg Press: This machine works your quads, glutes, hamstrings, and calves. Are you having trouble with good bodyweight squats? Use this machine as a trainer. Just like with a standing squat, push through your heels to extend weight. Think of your belly button being pulled to your spine to keep your core tight and form a flat belly rather than a rounded barrel belly.

Hamstring Curl: Isolate your hamstrings to work them out with this machine. It's a great machine for people who are new to resistance training and helps ensure that your quads don't become stronger than your hamstrings.

Cable Machine: This machine allows you to perform a variety of exercises, including biceps curls, triceps pushdowns, weighted abs curl, single-arm cable rows, etc.

Free Weights

What's great about free weights is that you can add them to a lot of the bodyweight resistance moves to up the resistance factor. You already have the form down – just add weight. Your form is sometimes slightly different when you add weight so pay close attention to the variation.

Proper Form Prevents Injury

One of the biggest disadvantages of free weights is the possibility of injury. Therefore, it is essential to use excellent form with every move. It is a good idea to practice the proper form with low or no weight (just the bar) until you can perform the move correctly.

Proper Weight

You are lifting the correct weight when you can do ten repetitions, with the last two coming with quite a bit of effort. When you can perform all ten with ease, it is time to add weight.

Adding Weight

When and How

When ten repetitions come easily, it is time to add weight. You should be able to do eight repetitions while putting in a lot of effort on the last two repetitions. Add weights five pounds at a time to increase your weight until you are doing eight repetitions, with two more being difficult – but not impossible – to do.

How to Know if You've Added Too Much

If you feel seriously strained when you lift a weight, if you cannot make ten repetitions, if you are seriously sore the next day, you have done too much weight. Cut back. Follow the guidelines above to know when and how to add weight. Ten repetitions is a good number of reps to shoot for. Add weight if you can easily do more reps. Cut back on weight if you can only do eight reps.

Sample Free Weight Routine

Perform full-body exercises and larger muscle exercises, like squats, before smaller movement, smaller muscle exercises like bicep curls.

Weighted Glute Bridge: This is a great exercise for your glutes (butt), hamstrings, and calves.

- Lie on your back with knees bent and feet flat on the floor.
- Place a dumbbell over your hips, keeping it in the same place without moving with your hands. You can put a towel under it for comfort.
- Tighten your core and keep it tight throughout this move. Pushing through your heels as you do when you rise in a squat, thrust your hips skyward until you are straight from knees to shoulders.
- Pause.
- Release in a controlled motion back down until butt bounces on the ground.
- Repeat.

Weighted Lunge: Quads, hamstrings, glutes, and calves all get worked as you perform a lunge while holding a barbell in each hand hanging at your hips.

- Step forward on one foot while your other foot is balanced on toes.
- Bend back leg until the knee touches the ground.
- Lift yourself back up.
- Switch legs.
- This exercise can be repeated with one leg forward for the intended number of reps (8-15) and then the other or switching legs with each rise.

Barbell Back Squat: Squats are an amazing exercise. They work so many muscles in your body that if you combine them with bench press and deadlift, you have a whole body workout in just three moves. This move is going to work your butt, your front and back thighs, your inner thighs – which are difficult to work – your hip flexors, your calves, your abs, and your lower back. Wow! Just wow! Let's get to it.

- Perfect your squat with bodyweight resistance before you add weight. Then start with a low weight. Even just a barbell is fine. Make sure you are still performing the move perfectly. Then – and only then – are you ready to add weight.
- Load the barbell onto your shoulders from a squat rack.
- With good squat form, sit back in your hips, bending your knees as though you are sitting back onto a chair. Keep your chest up and your eyes focused ahead of you.
- Sit until your thighs are parallel to the ground.
- When your thighs are parallel, your butt is dipped low, push through your heels to return to standing. Do this with *strength,* not momentum.
- Repeat.

Bench Press: Amazing move number two. Combined with Squats and Deadlift, you've got a three-move whole-body workout. This move works your entire chest, especially that glamour muscle (the pecs) that gives you a broad-chested, 'manly' look. It also works your arms and your upper back. Here's how to do it:

- Lie flat on your back on the bench.
- Grip the bar with hands slightly more than shoulder-width apart.
- Inhale as you bring the bar slowly down to your chest.
- As you exhale, push the bar, focusing your eyes on the ceiling, until your arms are extended but not locked.
- In a controlled manner, lower the bar back to your chest but do not rest it on your body.
- When you've finished your repetitions, rerack holding onto the bar until you are sure the bar is secure.

Deadlift: Remember I said you could combine squats with two other moves for a whole-body workout in just three moves? This is move number three. This doubles on hamstrings, glutes, and lower back, plus it works your upper back. Use a light pair of weights until you are sure you've got excellent form.

- Stand behind the barbell with your feet shoulder-width apart.
- Hinge at the waist, keeping your back straight.
- Bend your knees and grip the barbell.
- Roll your shoulders down and back.
- As you inhale, straighten your legs to lift the barbell as you unhinge your hips.
- To lower the barbell, hinge at your hips and control the movement to the ground.
- Repeat.
  - **Thruster:** You can replace the deadlift with this move and even get in a little cardio. It's a combination of a front squat and an overhead press.
- With feet shoulder-width apart, hold the barbell in an overhand grip with hands shoulder-width apart.
- Shoulders should be back and down with an aligned spine and slightly bent knees.
- Bring the barbell to your collarbone with your elbows facing forward. Your core should be engaged.
- Expand your chest, keeping core engaged as you lower your body into a deep squat. Knees should be slightly turned out.
- Press heels into the floor and bring your elbows up to explode upwards back to the stand.
- Press bar overhead.
- Bring the bar back to your shoulders in a controlled motion.
- Lower barbell to hips.
- Repeat the entire sequence.

Overhead Shoulder Press: For your deltoids, chest, triceps, and traps. Keep torso tight throughout. If you have back strain or torso movement, spread your feet for a wider stance or lower weight. Remember, your form is important to prevent injury.

- Stand with feet shoulder-width or slightly wider apart and a dumbbell in each hand at shoulder height with palms facing out.
- Press dumbbells upward until arms are fully extended. Pause.
- Return arms to shoulders in a slow and controlled manner.
- Repeat 8-15 reps.

Single-Arm Dumbbell Row: This is for most of your back, your biceps and triceps, and your *Erector Spinae* (the muscle responsible for keeping your spine aligned correctly). Here we go:

- Brace your arm on the back of a chair or a bench. The lower your hand, the more resistance you will get from the weight, and the harder your workout will be. You can place your knee on the bench if you're lifting a heavier weight.
- Grasp the dumbbell in the non-bracing hand.
- Pull the dumbbell up towards your chest, keeping your elbow tight against your body, until your upper arm is just beyond horizontal.
- Lower in a controlled manner - *do not drop weight* – until arm is extended and shoulder is stretched down.
- Repeat 8 – 15 reps.
- Switch arms and supporting arm/leg.

Floor Press: Can't get on a bench? This is a chest press on the ground. It's great for beginners to learn the proper feel for a bench press because you can feel your shoulders and back engaging as you do the press.

- Lie on your back with knees bent and feet flat on the floor.

- With a dumbbell in each hand, put your arms out to the sides of your body at a 45-degree angle and the dumbbells in the air.
- Push the dumbbells up on an exhale while you are extending your arms.
- Pause and hold at the top.
- Return in a controlled movement until your elbows touch the ground.
- Repeat 8-15 times.

Resistance Bands

Proper form prevents injury

Not only does proper form prevent injury to your muscles with resistance bands, but you can actually have injuries related to the band itself if you do not perform with proper form with these. Follow instructions accurately.

Resistance bands give you as much of a workout as weights of the same strength, don't hesitate to use them. The advantages are that they are inexpensive and highly portable and this means they travel well. They give you a completely different workout than any other form of resistance training and variety from your other workouts as well. Try resistance bands today.

Proper resistance

Bands come in several different levels, for example, light, medium, heavy, and very heavy. Buy at least three because you will need different weights depending on the muscle group you are working. You may only want a lightweight to work your wrist, but a very heavyweight may be necessary when you go to work your body through squats.

You will also find that they come with or without accessories. Use them according to your personal preference.

Adding resistance - When and How

When ten repetitions come easily, it is time to add weight. You should be able to do eightrepetitions while putting in effort on the last two repetitions. Move to the next heavier band when you can complete eight easy repetitions. When that band becomes too easy, move to the next heavier band.

How to Know if You've Added Too Much

As with other resistance training, if you are seriously sore the next day, you have added too much weight. Move back to a less heavy band.

Sample Resistance Band Exercises for Strength

Overhead Squat: Remember that technique is the most important part of this exercise. Put your feet into the band to anchor it to the ground, putting the band right under your arch. Spread your feet slightly more than shoulder-width apart. Squat into the band gripping it in your palms with the band wrapped to the outside of your hips and shoulders and your fists next to your shoulders. Stand tall, stretching your arms above your head. This is your starting position.

- Drop your butt down until you are bent 90° at the knee. As you come down, if you see your hands, your hands are too far forward. Keep them right overhead, as this forces you to drop your butt down.
- Press back up.
- Repeat.

The Bent-Over Row: Anchor your body the same way you did for the squat. Widen your stance. Grip the band on the outside near your knees, lower for more resistance, higher for less resistance. Keep your back flat or slightly arched, chin up.

- Pull elbows out wide, squeezing your shoulders together as though you were squeezing a tennis ball between your shoulder blades.
- *Variation:* With a lighter resistance band, or doubling the band for more resistance, place the whole band beneath your feet so that you have a loop sticking out from each foot. Wrap the band around your wrists. Now pull your elbows out wide as instructed above.
  - **Biceps Curl**: Anchor under the soles of your feet with feet hip-width apart. With arms turned out, palms facing away from your body, grip band with thumbs down.
- Curl up, keeping pinkies high – don't let your thumbs pivot up, keep them out. Lower back down. The band keeps constant tension on your arms.

Triceps: Wrap the band around an anchor at about waist height by thrusting one end through the loop of another end.

- Stand with one leg bent, step back on the other. Lean forward until your body is parallel to the ground.
- Grasp the band with the opposite arm from the forward foot. Your elbow will stay fixed with your upper arm aligned at your side.
- Thrust forearm back until fully extended.
- Slowly return to 90°.
- Remember that your elbow remains fixed at your side throughout exercise.
  - *Variation*: If you cannot anchor onto something, kneel on the ground and hitch your thumb through the loop of the band. Place your hand with the band extended forward onto the ground in front of you - centered to your body. Now grasp the band with your other hand and perform as above.

- o **Banded Push up**: Put your hands, flat palmed, through each side of the band with it low across the back of your shoulders. Drop into planking position and perform a push up. Keep the band anchored towards your palm rather than your fingers. Perform slow, controlled reps. Remember, you are now performing your push ups *with weight.*
- o **Standing Shoulder Press:** Set up as for Overhead Squat.
- Elbows straight out to the side. Press straight overhead.
- Return hands to shoulders. Repeat
  - o **Single-Leg Calf Raise**: Hook the band under the toe of one foot and over the shoulder of the same arm. Put toes on a half-brick or weight plate.
- Press up.
- Lower heel.
- Repeat.

Band Crunch: Loop Band around an anchor. Assume basic crunch position with head at the band. Hold one side of the band in each hand. Put the base of palms at the sides of the head.

- Crunch head gently towards knees lifting shoulders in a curl off of the mat. This is only a slight curl that crunches your abs. Because you're holding onto the band, you are adding weight to your crunch, and this means you are getting a much heavier workout than if you do it without the band.

See-Saw: You've been doing most of your workout alone. Here's a chance for you to buddy up and have some partner fun. This move strengthens your lower body, your core, and your upper body – in both of you. Remember that partnering for your workout can keep you from dropping out because your partner expects you to be there – it's one of those social pressure moves that keep you doing something simply because it's what's expected of you. Sometimes peer pressure is a good thing. Here's how to do the resistance band see-saw:

- Both partners hold the band overhead with both hands. Make the band taut between you and keep it taut throughout the exercise.
- Partner A squats with the band between the legs, arms straight, band tight.
- Partner B stands with arms lifted high overhead, arms straight, band tight.
- As the first partner, Partner A, stands and lifts their arms overhead, Partner B will then shift to a squat, lowering hands between the legs.
- The movement should imitate a playground see-saw.
    - Keep the band taut at all times.
    - Keep arms straight at throughout the movement.
    - Do not arch your back.
    - Squat properly with feet slightly wider than hip-distance. Bend at the knees, hinging at the hips as though sitting onto a chair behind you. When rising, press through the heels.
    - Keep core straight and tight at all times.

Sample Resistance Band Exercises for Cardio/Aerobics

Seated Row: Sit on the floor with legs straight out. Wrap the band around your feet. As your hands are stretched towards your feet, the band should have some resistance.

- Keep your back straight.
- Lean back slightly.
- Bend knees slightly.
- Pull elbows back until hands are at your chest.
- In a controlled manner, release back to start.
- Repeat.

Resistance Push Ups: This exercise is the same as the banded push up exercise above. *Variation to Increase Difficulty:* Support feet on a bench – the higher the bench, the more difficult. Now perform the same move.

Standing Lateral Raises: Stand over the band with your feet shoulder-width apart. Hold the band in each hand with your palms facing your legs.

- Lift your arms either at the same time or alternating out to the side until they are parallel to the ground.
- Return to side.
- This is a controlled, steady movement focusing on your shoulders.
- Repeat as many times as possible in one minute to make it aerobic.
- Rest for 30 seconds.

Lunges: Anchor the band under one foot. Step back with the other. Hold the band in each hand just under your chin.

- Bend your back knee to touch the ground, keeping the front knee behind your toe.
- This works your quadriceps, hamstrings, and glutes.
- Rise in a nice controlled manner.
- Repeat as many times as you can with good form in one minute.
- Rest for 30 seconds.

Standing Press Squat: Remember that technique is the most important part of this exercise. Put your feet into the band to anchor it to the ground, putting the band right under your arch. Spread your feet slightly more than shoulder-width apart. Squat into the band gripping it in your palms with the band wrapped to the outside of your hips and shoulders and your fists next to your shoulders. Stand tall, stretching your arms above your head. This is your starting position.

- Drop your butt down until you are bent 90° at the knee. As you come down, if you see your hands, your hands are too far forward. Keep them right overhead, and this forces you to drop your butt down.
- Press back up.
- Lower arms to your waist.
- Press arms back overhead.
- Repeat the entire sequence.
- Perform as many well-controlled reps as possible in one minute.
- Rest for 30 seconds.

Resisted Boxer: Anchor the band. Some bands come with a loop you attach to a doorknob or other anchor point, you loop through itself with the doubled other end. Hold handles or looped end in each hand.

- Step forward with one foot. Extend opposite arm in front of the chest as though punching, palm down.
- Switch arms while jumping to switch legs at the same time.
- Add more resistance by standing further from the anchor point. Add even more resistance with a heavier band.
- Keep breath steady and even while repeating as many as possible for one minute before resting for 30 seconds. Resume the exercise and keep going.

Squat Hops with Press Back: Use the same anchored band. Stand facing anchor while holding the band with arms hanging at sides of the body with palms facing back. There will be moderate tension on the band. Feet should be slightly more than hip-width apart.

- Squat with good form while pressing arms back towards hips and stretching band.
- Push through heels with energy, launching yourself into the air while bringing arms forward in front of the chest.

- Land in the squat position.
- Press arms back.
- Repeat quickly with good form as many times as possible in one minute.
- Rest for 30 seconds.
- Add more resistance by standing further from the anchor point. Add even more resistance with a heavier band.

Standing Swim: Use the same anchored band. Stand facing the anchor point with feet hip-width apart, and have your knees slightly bent, band in hands with arms down at sides. Your core will remain tight and engaged throughout the movement.

- Raise one arm and 'swim' backward as in the backstroke. Allow the body to turn slightly with the movement. Complete rotation and begin the same movement with the other arm.
- Alternate the movement between each side as quickly as possible, maintaining good form for one minute.
- Rest for 30 seconds.
- Add more resistance by standing further from the anchor point. Add even more resistance with a heavier band.

Skating Squats: Stand inside the band, anchoring it under the soles of your feet. Your feet should be about hip-width apart. Grip band with elbows bent at your waist. There should be full resistance in this position.

- Lower into a perfect squat.
- As you rise quickly out of your squat, extend one leg to the side.
- Step down onto that leg and back into the squat.
- Raise quickly again, lifting the opposite leg.
- Alternate side as quickly as possible for one minute.
- Rest for 30 seconds.

- Add more resistance by standing further from the anchor point. Add even more resistance with a heavier band.

Moving Twister: This works your obliques as well as giving you cardio. Use your band anchored at chest height. Face it and grasp it in both hands.

- Skip to the side two steps.
- Swing both arms to the side that you shuffled towards.
- Shuffle to the other side.
- Swing both arms to the side that you shuffled towards.
- Alternate side as quickly as possible for one minute.
- Rest for 30 seconds.
- Add more resistance by standing further from the anchor point. Add even more resistance with a heavier band.

Chest Punch: You will work your chest, shoulder, triceps, obliques, and core. Use the same shoulder-height, anchored band.

- Stand with one foot forward and balance on the toes of the back foot where you will be pivoting.
- Punch forward with the arm on the side of the pivoting leg twisting as you thrust across your body.
- Repeat 15 times before switching sides.

Upward Wood Chop: Attach the band to a low point. Stand with the band on the outside of your foot and reach down to grasp it in both hands.

- Pull up and across your body as you pivot, bringing hands to the opposite side of the body to just above head height.
- This works shoulders, core, and legs.
- *Variation:* Bend knee as in a lunge and raise all the way up.
- Repeat 10-15 times per side.

Downward Wood Chop: Attach the band to a high point. Stand with the band on the outside of your shoulder and reach up to grasp it in both hands.

- Pull down and across your body as you pivot, bringing hands to the opposite side of the body to just below hip height. Keep your arms locked.
- This works shoulders, core, and legs.
- Repeat 10-15 times per side.

Cool Down

A cool-down after your exercise allows your heart rate to return to normal while your breathing also becomes deeper and returns to normal, if not slower. Your body will continue to burn extra calories for as much as 24 hours. The cool-down allows your muscles to slowly return to a normal temperature and all of the 'feel-good' hormones and chemicals (like dopamine and serotonin) to slowly return to a normal state.

Studies have shown that cooling down prevents your body from cramping as well. This is especially important after strength training when your muscles are more likely to suffer from soreness. Since your muscles are still warm, this is a good time to add some flexibility into your routine with gentle stretching as you return your body to its pre-workout state.

Flexibility is good for every part of your life. When you are flexible, your reflexes react more quickly as they do not have to resist the pull of your stiff muscles. When you are flexible, you can be more active in bed. Since you're exercising more, your testosterone levels can increase, and tis means you are more likely to want to have more sex. Therefore, you will *want* to be able to perform better, more actively, in bed. Exercising and stretching will help you do that. So for sex's sake – stretch!

Overhead Stretch: This barely needs instruction. You do it naturally almost every day. Stretch your arms overhead. As you get older, this becomes more and more difficult. But you will find that right after a workout, when your muscles are nice and warm, it's not so tough and it is a good flexibility stretch to maintain youthfulness. Lift your hands and reach up, grasp your wrists together, and make yourself taller. Allow the stretch to run from your fingers down the length of your arms. Stretch your spine up and feel a lengthening from your neck all the way down to your toes. Hold for ten to twenty seconds as you slightly pulse with your hands past your head. For variety, you can lean slightly to the right then slowly lean to the left. Stretch back to the center. Lower your arms and allow them to swing at your sides for another ten to twenty seconds. Repeat. Do this five or more times. This exercise can help you resist the aging pull of gravity.

Biceps Stretch: Raise both arms overhead. Bend left arm at the elbow. Use the right hand to gently stretch your left elbow back, creating a gentle stretch in your bicep. Hold for 20 seconds. Switch arms and perform this stretch on the other side for 20 seconds.

Wrist extensors: Stretch both arms out in front of you. Turn one arm palm up. Use the other hand to gently stretch the fingers of that hand down. Be very gentle as you do not want to rip any tendons. Hold gently for 20 seconds. Switch hands.

Wrist Rolls: This one looks pretty cool while you're doing it. Your grandkids will get a kick out of it. Interlace your fingers together in front of your chest. Rotate your hands in a circular motion rolling left over right then right over left. Continue in this direction for 30 seconds to a minute. Reverse the direction of the movement.

Doorway Stretch: This is especially good after bench press. Stand in an open doorway with each arm bent at a 90° angle with palms and elbows resting on the door frame. Step forward with one foot to press chest through the door frame feeling the stretch in shoulders and chest. Hold for 20 seconds or so. Repeat several times.

Sumo Squat Stretch: This is good for the groin and inner thigh (and therefore good for sex) and important after squat workouts, running workouts, any workouts that involve lots of lower bodywork.

- Stand with feet slightly more than hip-distance, just like for any other squat.
- Do your best squat.
- Put your hands between your knees and press out with your elbows.
- Hold.

Standing Lunge: Step one foot forward in a nice lunge position. Both feet should be flat on the ground. Twist your hips to the waist. Push forward with hips and back thigh stretching hips, ankles, and calves. Hold for thirty seconds to one minute. Switch sides.

Standing Calf Stretch: You can easily move into this stretch from the Standing Lunge by bending the back knee and shifting your weight onto the front heel. Now lean forward, bending at the waist, stretching your arms towards your extended front leg. Hold. As you exhale, allow your body to ease down into the stretch. Inhale and exhale slowly, stretching further with each exhale. Repeat on the other side. As with other stretches, as you continue to incorporate this into your daily workout, your stretch will get longer and further down.

Forward Bend: Another one that barely needs instruction. This stretches your hamstrings, calves, and even your back. Here's what's important to remember – rise *slowly*. You've just completed an intense workout. The blood is still racing through your body. In your cool down, you need to be aware of that manic blood flow and move accordingly. If you rise too quickly, you might cause yourself some lightheadedness or dizziness. You might even faint. So slow and steady is the rule.

- Roll forward from the waist one vertebrae at a time, allowing the weight of your arms, head, and then torso to pull your upper body down until you are touching your hands to the ground. Don't worry if your hands do not meet the ground. Simply follow the instructions.
- Inhale.
- As you exhale, relax into the stretch. You will feel it in your back from your neck over your spine and buttocks, down your hamstrings, all the way to your ankles.
- Inhale.
- As you exhale, relax further into the stretch allowing your body to pull you deeper towards your feet. This is why it doesn't matter if the first attempts did not bring your hands to your toes. With each exhale, it will relax you down further. It may take weeks for you to get to your toes, but if you incorporate this stretch into your cool-down routine every day, you will eventually get there.

Variation: Spread your legs farther than hip distance. Bend to one side. Stretch arms to the ankle and hold. Exhale and stretch further. Hold. Exhale and stretch. Continue this pattern for several rounds of breathing. Switch to the other side and repeat.

Seated Forward Bend: Sit with your legs extended straight in front of you. Reach your arms to your toes. You will feel the stretch from your shoulders all the way down your back, around your buttocks, under your legs, all the way to your ankles. If you cannot reach your toes, inhale and on the exhale, allow your body to relax farther down.

Don't 'stretch'. Simply relax further down. Inhale. Relax again farther with each exhale. If you experience too much tension in your back or hamstrings, bend your knees slightly but continue to relax your entire body farther into the stretch with each exhale. If you make this stretch a regular part of your cool down after every workout, you will find that after a week or two, your legs will become straighter, and you will be able to press your chest closer to your legs and your fingers closer to your toes.

Seated Twist: This stretches your hips and back. Sit with your legs extended straight in front of you. Cross the right leg over the left, bending the knee so your right foot sits flat on the ground. Place your right-hand flat on the ground behind you. Lift your chest as you turn your body to the right and place your left elbow over your right knee, stretching your knee and hip towards you gently. Hold as you inhale. As you exhale, allow the stretch to increase. Continue to inhale and exhale for about 10 seconds before slowly releasing and switching sides to repeat the stretch.

Lower Back Rotation Stretch: Lie on your back with your knees bent and your toes on the ground. With your shoulders remaining flat against the ground, rotate your knees as far to the side as you can. Hold, keeping your abdominals tight. Return to the center. Lower to the opposite side. Hold. Repeat. Hold for the same amount of time to each side, feeling the stretch on the outside of your thigh each time. With time, this stretch will eventually allow you to lower your legs to the ground. This is another stretch that directly benefits sex.

Bretzel Stretch: This is a full-body stretch. Lie on your side with a pillow or rolled-up towel under your neck (optional).

- Bend your top leg and bring it towards your chest until it's just slightly more than 90°.

- Grip it with your bottom hand.
- Bend your lower leg back and grasp your ankle with your top hand or use a towel or strap around that ankle to pull the leg backward.
- Inhale. Relax.
- Exhale as you slowly rotate your top shoulder back towards the ground.
- Inhale and relax.
- As you exhale, allow the shoulder to lift slightly, while pressing out with the bottom leg while moving the knee back and increasing the lower leg stretch.
- Inhale and relax shoulder back down.
- With each exhale, increase the stretch.
- Continue to exhale and stretch for one to three minutes.
- Release. Roll to the other side. Repeat the entire sequence.

As you make this stretch a more regular part of your workout, you will find that you can stretch your leg more easily behind you and lower your shoulder more fully to the mat as the days pass and your flexibility increases.

Core Abdominal Stretch: Also known as Cobra Pose. Lie on your stomach with your arms palms down at your chest. Lift your head and chest stretching up and back. Stretch as high as is comfortable for you. As with many stretches, the more often you perform this stretch, the further you will be able to go. Hold for a good long stretch.

Child's Pose: From all fours, extend your toes and sit back on your heels, letting your arms stretch out in front of you. Your stomach will rest on your thighs, and your head will rest on the ground between your arms. There will be tension along your spine and through your arms. With each exhale, allow your body to relax down into the stretch. Close your eyes and relax. *Variation*: Bring your arms alongside your body. This is less of a stretch but is still relaxing and a good final cool-down pose.

Legs Up the Wall Pose: Sit with the side of your body next to a wall. Swing your legs up the wall as you lie down on your back. Wiggle until your hips are against the wall or just a few inches away. Relax your arms on your stomach or over your head.

Other ways to Recover After a Workout:

- Drink Plenty of Fluids
- Massage
- Foam Roller Massage – this is a way to massage yourself.
- Ice Bath
- Steam Room
- Warm Soak in a Hot Bath
- Aqua Massage

CHAPTER 4: INJURY

Injury Prevention and Recovery

You must do everything possible to *avoid* injury. That means proper technique first and foremost. It also means proper gear. And it means increasing resistance and distance by slow and appropriate increments. Be certain you *start* every workout with a warm-up and *end* every workout with a cool down. If you consistently follow these rules, you should be able to avoid injury most of the time.

Unfortunately, injuries aren't always avoidable. When the ill-fated does occur, do everything you can to recover as quickly as possible. But do not restart your workout routine until you are fully recovered. Pain is an indicator of injury. Let your body's pain be your guide.

The most common types of injuries are:

- Sprains to ankle and wrist
- Muscle Strains
- Tendinitis
- Meniscus and ACL tears of the knee
- Rotator Cuff Tears

Injury Recovery

You want to avoid injury at all possible costs. Using the proper form in all that you do is the best way to do that. You don't have *time* for an injury.

Take your downtime to examine how and why you were injured in the first place. Did you push yourself too far? Lift too much weight before you were ready? Was there social pressure moving you to do so? Most importantly, were you using the proper technique. This is *the most important* injury prevention method available to you.

Your First response – R.I.C.E: Rest-Ice-Compression-Elevation. Your first response to an injury should be to immediately cease working out and give your injured area a rest. Ice the area of injury, although some injuries respond better to heat. Compress if possible. Obviously, that's not a good idea with a neck injury. Elevate your injury to get the blood to flow away from the injury that helps to decrease inflammation.

If your pain is so intense that you cannot sit still, or you are moaning in pain, call an ambulance, or have someone immediately drive you to a hospital. Otherwise, use the above procedure for two or three days. Generally speaking, the swelling increases over the first 24 hours. Then you should see lessening with ice and compression. It's important to apply RICE from the beginning to lessen the amount of swelling. Ibuprofen or another anti-inflammatory pain medication can also help with both pain and inflammation.

When to see your doctor - If your pain is so intense that you cannot sit still, or you are moaning in pain, call an ambulance, or have someone immediately drive you to a hospital.

If pain and swelling haven't seen some improvement in two days, see your doctor. X-rays or MRI may be needed depending on the extent of injury and location. If the injury is severe, therapy such as physical therapy may be needed. Follow your doctor's advice.

When and How to resume your routine – Once your injury has healed to the point that your doctor has given you clearance, or you can put weight on it if you did not need to see a doctor, you can resume a gentle program. Do not dive right back into the weights you were lifting or the aerobic capacity you were doing at the time of the injury.

You took your downtime to examine *why* you were injured. Use that knowledge to adjust your needs to prevent injury. Did you push yourself too far? Then you need to cut well back on your routine. Increase your workout incrementally, and if you feel sore beyond one day's recovery, you have gone too far. Don't do that same extension in your next workout. Add a smaller increment.

Was there social pressure pushing you to increase your weight or distance to the level that caused your injury? Do not cave in to it. If the temptation is too great, choose different workout partners or workout alone. Your body is your temple. You cannot afford to lose it. It is more fragile after 50 and takes greater care and longer to recover. You cannot compete with men in their 30s. Do not attempt to do so. They will recover much more quickly than you. They also may cause permanent damage to their body with an injury that they will have to live with for 20 more years than you.

To prevent another injury, be certain that you use the correct technique. That applies to activities such as walking, hiking, and jogging as well. Start with a warm-up and end with a cool down.

You need to wear shoes that support your feet properly and give you good impact resistance so that you don't develop shin splints and other related injuries. Consult with a shoe expert for appropriate footwear in stores such as Runner's Warehouse and REI, which carry a wide variety of athletic shoes.

Remember, your first defense is prevention. Use proper technique but understand that injury isn't always avoidable.

CHAPTER 5: DIET

Why Healthy Diets Are More Crucial Than Ever After the Age of 50.

You already know that it is harder to maintain weight after the age of 50. We gain weight at 1 to 2 pounds per year every year past 30 unless we work diligently to counteract that process. We lose muscle as we age. We lose the hormones that keep us muscular, and we tend to store fat over muscle. All those factors cause us to tend to put on weight and to have a higher fat percentage of our body weight.

To stop that from happening, exercise is essential. But so is a healthy diet. You've seen your physician, and you've discussed your health with him/her. If you have dietary restrictions, follow those guidelines first and foremost. If you do not, you will find healthy eating guidelines in this chapter.

No need to moan. You can maintain a healthy weight and still eat a delicious diet now that you are exercising and generating muscle. Don't pay attention to fad diets that tell you you can never eat a single carb. Or that you have to drink only protein shakes. Or that wheat germ, soy, and tofu are the only foods that can ever pass your lips again. None of that is true. Even fasting is just a fad.

You can eat a normal, healthy diet as long as you continue to keep up your exercise routine. What does that mean? Well, it means 'moderation in all things.' You can have something sweet now and then. But not every day. You can have a little salt. But you can't overdo it. You can have carbs – but not *just* carbs. You need to balance it out with protein.

You've been doing more strength training than ever before. Maintaining muscle requires protein. Therefore, the healthy diet for the person who strength-trains needs to include plenty of protein. Find protein in meats (avoid processed meats), cheeses, eggs, milk, and nuts.

You need to eat a well-balanced, well-rounded diet. To help you out, there's one outlined below.

Healthy Diet

Here are a couple of basic guidelines to pay attention to now that you're over 50:

- Eat more fiber: Try to get 20 - 30 grams of fiber per day.
- Cut down on salt: limit salt intake to 1,500 milligrams (2/3 teaspoon) per day.
- Stay hydrated: For a man, that means 15 ½ cups or 3.7 liters of fluid (such as water, or juice – does not include caffeinated or alcoholic drinks) per day.

Sample Healthy Diet

- Breakfast –
  - o 1/2 cup Fiber One Cereal - You've just eaten more than half of your body's daily requirement of fiber. Good job!
  - o ½ Cup 2% Milk on cereal
  - o Juice, Coffee, or Water (The caffeine in coffee is good for sharpening your memory. Drink it with cream to keep your sugar intake to a minimum.)
- Snack –
  - o Water
  - o Whole Wheat Avocado Toast (you just ate some more fiber)
  - o Or
  - o Apple Slices with Carmel Dip (See how versatile this can be?)

- Lunch –
- ○ Steak Fajita Power Bowl
    - ○ Fry up fajita vegetables in olive oil. Set aside.
    - ○ Sauté flank steak with cumin, chili powder, and a dash of salt until cooked through. Save some flank steak for steak tacos tonight.
    - ○ Place ingredients over brown rice with corn, black beans, and avocado. Top with a bit of sour cream and cilantro. (That brown rice has fiber, btw.)
- **Snack** – This is a high magnesium snack with flavonoids to lower the risk of heart disease and monounsaturated fats that are beneficial for blood sugar control. This snack will fill you up, feed your sugar craving, and keep your heart healthy. Depending on the cocoa content, you should be around 300 calories.
    - ○ One ounce dark chocolate
    - ○ Handful of almonds
- Dinner –
    - ○ Fajita Tacos – You saved some fajita steak from lunch. Use it to make some delicious tacos.
    - ○ Top with Guacamole as avocados provide vitamins C, E, K, and B-6, as well as numerous additional nutrients. Most of their fat comes from monounsaturated fatty acids that are good for you.
    - ○ Feel free to add sour cream and cheese for the protein benefits.
    - ○ There's absolutely nothing negative about salsa. Add lots.
    - ○ Feel free to have a glass of wine with this meal as wine has antioxidants that help improve memory, protect against heart disease, and decrease inflammation. Those who follow a Mediterranean diet that includes wine with evening meals have been shown to live longer and suffer fewer incidences of Alzheimer's.

Losing Weight

If you need to lose a drastic amount of weight, consult a dietician and/or your doctor. If you simply wish to lose a few pounds and you have not exercised until now, give your new exercise program about four weeks combined with the healthy eating guidelines described above. You will probably find that is all you need to begin to lose weight.

Remember, fat requires less energy for the body to operate than muscle. You're putting on muscle that will burn more calories, causing your body to begin to drop weight.

If you need to lose more weight, below is a sample of a 1200 calorie diet. Be certain that you drink the recommended amount of water, as outlined at the beginning of this chapter. High fiber is especially important. Drink coffee or tea as well. However, do not add sugar or cream as this will up your caloric intake. Finally, try to eat slowly. This will allow your food to hit your stomach and register as 'full' before you finish your meal.

Sample Weight Loss Diet

- Breakfast –
  - 1/2 cup Fiber One Cereal - You've just eaten more than half of your body's daily requirement of fiber. Good job!
  - 1 Cup Fat-free Milk on cereal
  - One banana – you can have this on your cereal or separate
  - Coffee or tea or water, or all three (The caffeine in coffee is good for sharpening your memory. Drink it with only cream to keep your sugar intake to a minimum.)
- Lunch –
  - Fill a whole-wheat pita with 3 oz turkey breast, ½ roasted pepper, 1 tsp mayonnaise, a dab of mustard, and lettuce.

- o One stick part-skim mozzarella string cheese
- o Your choice of fruit (more fiber!)
- Dinner –
  - o Four ounces broiled flounder with sliced plum tomatoes sprinkled with two tablespoons grated parmesan cheese.
  - o 1 cup cooked couscous
  - o 1 cup steamed broccoli
- Desert
  - o Single Serve Ice Cream – yes, you get a treat. If you feel entirely deprived, you won't stick with it.

Gaining Weight

If you're one of the lucky few who need to gain weight, this diet is for you. There are a few guidelines to follow to make it easier for you to put on some pounds, and then there is a calorie-rich sample diet to follow.

- Eat frequently. Just like with losing or maintaining weight, in order to gain weight, frequent meals can be the key. You may feel full quickly. Eating frequent meals allows you to eat more calories than if you only eat three meals. Try eating six meals a day instead. If each of these meals contains as many calories as your three-meal plan, you will be eating twice as many calories with the same amount of intake at each sitting.
- Avoid drinking for 30 minutes before your meals. Sip a high-calorie drink during your meal but nothing bubbly as this may make you feel full quicker, and this could prevent you from eating your full caloric intake.
- Instead of drinking diet soda, coffee, and other lower-calorie beverages between meals, try consuming heavier calorie drinks such as smoothies or shakes. Milk is also a good choice. Studies show that milk leads to greater mass gain than other protein sources. See the sample diet below for milk smoothies.

- Snack on high calorie, nutritious foods such as nuts, peanut butter, cheese, dried fruit, avocadoes, and meats.
- Have treats. Excess sugar should always be monitored, but an occasional treat such as ice cream or dark chocolate is an acceptable treat - especially treats like dark chocolate that has flavonoids and antioxidants that help with inflammation and memory.
- Remember that exercise will put muscle on your body, especially strength training. Choose muscle building exercises for your cardio/aerobic workouts like calisthenics.

Sample Diet

- Breakfast:
- Milk Smoothy:
- One cup frozen berries of your choice
- One cup whole milk
- Two teaspoons honey
- One teaspoon vanilla

  Combine all ingredients in a blender until smooth and rich.

- Lunchtime:
- Smoked salmon – Eat your smoked salmon on whole grain bread with cream cheese, cucumber, tomato, and capers.
- Sliced avocado on the side – these are calorie-dense and they really help with weight gain. Eat them often as they are also loaded with vitamins, minerals, and various beneficial plant compounds.
- Rice with parmesan cheese.
- Broccoli
- Dinner:
- Smoked brisket

- Baked Potato loaded with butter, sour cream, bacon, chives, and cheese
- Corn
- Tossed salad with oil and vinegar dressing
- Warm rolls

Make the potato in an instant pot with the brisket for easy cooking. Slather everything you can in butter for extra calories. No low-calorie anything here. Use the full-calorie versions. No low fat either. You're trying to gain weight.

Cheese, milk, and eggs are great protein sources that also help you gain weight. Combine them (as in scrambled eggs), or eat them in combination with other weight gaining-foods such as potatoes. Add them to salads, casseroles, and sandwiches.

Add healthy fats and oils such as extra virgin olive oil, avocado oil, and coconut oil. Use them in your cooking.

You'll be gaining weight in no time.

Maintaining Weight

Beware of empty calories in things such as beer, sodas, snacks, desserts, even gum.

Sample Diet

Follow the diet example in **Healthy Diet** shown above. Be sure to consume the appropriate amounts of water, and to follow any dietary restrictions your doctor has suggested.

How to Prepare a Healthy Diet When You're Pressed for Time.

Precooking: Precooking is one of the quickest ways to clear up your schedule. Let's say you need a lean lunch. Cook three pieces of chicken in your instant pot. It only takes 10 minutes total – five minutes cooking and five minutes pressure release. Do it at whichever mealtime you have the most time, whether that's lunch or dinner. Now you have dinner chicken, lunch chicken, and lunch for another day as well. All with only one cooking. For the next two meals, you can either eat the chicken cold or zap it in the microwave.

Stir Fry: To make stir fry as fast as possible, follow these steps.

- Use a wok.
- Buy stir fry vegetables or julienned vegetables.
- Purchase pre-cut chicken.
- Use bottled stir fry sauce.
- Use a jar of minced garlic. (This also keeps your hands from getting smelly, cutting clean up time.)
- Use minute rice.
- Marinade chicken while you heat the wok.
- Add one tablespoon olive oil.
- Remove chicken from marinade (reserving the marinade) and add to wok, cooking thoroughly (about five minutes). Remove chicken and set aside.
- Boil water for rice.
- Add more olive oil if needed and add about one clove of minced garlic. Cook for about a minute.
- Add rice to water, and cover.
- Add vegetables until warmed.
- Add chicken and marinade back to the wok. Heat until thoroughly mixed and hot.

- Serve stir fry over rice.

Use a meal delivery service: There are several choices these days for having meals delivered to your home. You select meals from a menu every week, and the ingredients for a portioned meal arrive at your door. You don't have to take the time to shop for the food, only prepare it. A big time saver. Here are a couple of services to choose from:

- HelloFresh
- Blue Apron
- Fresh and Easy
- Every Plate
- Sun Basket
- Freshly
- Martha and Marley Spoon
- Nutrisystem
- Trifecta
- Dinnerly
- Home Chef
- Green Chef

Cookie Sheet Dinners: These are dinners that you toss together on a cookie sheet or in a baking dish, then shove in the oven for 20 to 45 minutes. Yes, it's really that simple. The preparation is next to nothing and you do your thing – your workout, for example, while dinner's cooking. Here are a couple of examples to get you started.

- Kielbasa and potatoes
  - Slice up your favorite pre-cooked *Kielbasa* into ¼ inch slices.
  - Slice two to three potatoes into bite-sized chunks (the size of the potato chunks determines the length of the cooking time).

- Toss potatoes and *Kielbasa* in olive oil.
- Slice onion into chunks similar to the size of potato chunks.
- Pour contents of one jar of mild banana peppers over *Kielbasa*, potatoes, and onions.
- Add several long sprigs of fresh basil. You will be removing these before serving.
- Cook in 425° oven for 45 minutes. The meal is done when the potatoes are soft.
  - Remove basil before serving.
- Roasted Shrimp and Polenta
  - Lightly coat pan with olive oil.
  - Slice polenta into ½" rounds.
  - Place polenta on the pan.
  - Toss a pint of halved cherry tomatoes in kosher salt, freshly ground pepper, and a teaspoon of olive oil.
  - Place on top of polenta, and place it in 400° oven for 10 minutes.
  - While that's cooking, mix 1 ½ Tablespoons olive oil with 1 tablespoon lemon juice, 1 clove minced (from a jar) garlic, ½ teaspoon oregano, ½ teaspoon Worcestershire sauce, salt and pepper, and chives. Once this is whisked together, toss the shrimp in it.
  - Put shrimp over the top of the polenta and tomatoes and cook an additional 10 minutes or until shrimp are pink and just cooked through.
- Meatloaf
  - Mix a pound of ground beef, a half tablespoon of dried mustard, a cup of bread crumbs, and an egg together and form into a loaf in a roasting pan.
  - Cover meatloaf with ketchup or gravy.
  - Surround meatloaf with new potatoes and carrots.
  - Cover with tinfoil.
  - Bake at 350° for about 45 minutes.

All these healthy meals come with a short preparation time to make life as simple as possible. Stick it in the oven and forget about it. You've got this.

CONCLUSION

Now that you're over 50, it's time to crack down. No more playing around. You have no more time to waste by leaving your health and fitness to chance. You simply must get to it. Every year you're losing muscle mass, and more of your physique is turning to flab. No more!

This book showed you how to change all that and get into the shape you need to be in for the rest of your fit life.

You're a busy man. You need results, and you want to see them quickly. This program will have you seeing *visible* results in as little as four weeks. And you'll feel more fit even sooner. All you have to do is put one foot in front of the other and start moving.

There are programs here for everyone, from the couch potato who hasn't moved in years to the athlete who just needs more motivation. And there's enough information to keep you interested day after day, week after week, month after month. Variety is what's going to keep you working at it. And that's what you need.

There are motivators here to make you want to hit the gym. Flip back through this awesome book to remind yourself just how to train and why you want to hit the gym – again!

Thank you for making it through to the end of *Fitness Over 50*. It's been able to provide you with all of the tools you need to achieve your goals, whatever they may be. Share this informative book with your friends.

The next step, if you haven't already, is to get out there and start working out.

Finally, if you found this book useful in any way, a review on Amazon is always appreciated!

CPSIA information can be obtained
at www.ICGtesting.com
Printed in the USA
LVHW051323040121
675400LV00006B/1119

9 781513 676937